WEIGHT WATCHERS
Family Power

WEIGHT WATCHERS
Family Power

5 Simple Rules for a Healthy-Weight Home

Karen Miller-Kovach

Foreword by Marc S. Jacobson, M.D.
Introduction by Meredith Vieira

WILEY

John Wiley & Sons, Inc.

Published by John Wiley & Sons, Inc., Hoboken, New Jersey
Published simultaneously in Canada

All photos by Gus Francisco Photography

Design and composition by Navta Associates, Inc.

The information contained in this book is not intended to serve as a replacement for professional medical advice. Any use of the information in this book is at the reader's discretion. The author and the publisher specifically disclaim any and all liability arising directly or indirectly from the use or application of any information contained in this book. A health care professional should be consulted regarding your specific situation.

For general information about our other products and services, please contact our Customer Care Department within the United States at (800) 762-2974, outside the United States at (317) 572-3993 or fax (317) 572-4002.

Wiley also publishes its books in a variety of electronic formats. Some content that appears in print may not be available in electronic books. For more information about Wiley products, visit our web site at www.wiley.com.

Library of Congress Cataloging-in-Publication Data:

Miller-Kovach, Karen.
  Weight Watchers family power : 5 simple rules for a healthy weight home / Karen Miller-Kovach ; foreword by Marc Jacobson, introduction by Meredith Vieira.
     p. cm.
  Includes bibliographical references and index.
  ISBN-13 978-0-471-77102-9 (cloth)
  ISBN-10 0-471-77102-3 (cloth)
  1. Children—Nutrition. 2. Family—Nutrition. 3. Parent and child. 4. Weight loss.
I. Title: Family power. II. Title.

RJ206.M687 2006
649'.3—dc22

                                                                    2005030512

Printed in the United States of America

10 9 8 7 6 5 4 3

Contents

Foreword

When I first read this book, I was overwhelmed with gratitude for the author, who has given us a clearly written guide we can use to navigate the issue of childhood overweight. We are facing a tremendous family health challenge—obesity. A growing number of children are overweight, as are their parents. Being too heavy increases a child's chances of facing major illness and leading a less healthy life.

Whether you are one of the millions of Weight Watchers members who needs help with a child in your family or a parent who has never struggled with your own weight but has a child with weight challenges, *Family Power: 5 Simple Rules for a Healthy-Weight Home* will give you enormous comfort, information, and help. The method recommended in this book takes into account what we've learned from the most advanced scientific studies available on overweight children combined with practical knowledge gained from decades of working with overweight adults. In my teaching of pediatricians, nutritionists, nurses, and others interested in children's health, I have touched on many of the points you will read here, but in this book the latest facts are clearly written and interlaced with real-world examples that you will find inspiring and instructive.

What is Family Power? It is the strength of parents, children, and other family members who work together as a team to improve the health of each and every person in the family. When it comes to family life, the whole is greater than the sum of the parts. Working together is more powerful and effective than working alone. Family Power is more important today than ever before.

In my practice as a pediatrician and a specialist in heart disease prevention in children, I am getting more and more referrals to work with children who have weight problems. This is not something that a child can or should deal with alone—a child needs the power of the family to guide and support him or her toward living a lifestyle that promotes healthy weight.

In this book you will read that parents truly need to understand the basics of weight management for children in order to help their children attain and maintain a healthy weight. My colleagues and I have researched what it takes to help a child be successful at maintaining a healthy weight (and, in our practice, improving heart health). The number one factor, we have discovered, is whether or not the parents get involved. Children whose parents play an active role in the health of the family become healthier. Playing an active role as a parent does not mean making changes just for the child. Parents need to change their own lifestyles by following the 5 Simple Rules that are so clearly described in part one of this book. These rules are easy to understand, they follow common-sense principles, and they apply to everyone in the household.

Parents may not realize just how much and in how many ways they influence their children every day. What parents eat, how they eat, and whether or not they are active have a huge effect. Part two of *Family Power: 5 Simple Rules for a Healthy-Weight Home* shows how parents play 5 different and essential roles that help their children to develop healthy habits. In describing each of the roles, the book guides parents through the small and gradual changes that they need to make to create a healthy-weight home for all family members.

A healthy-weight home and lifestyle are particularly important for children because kids are not mini-adults. That is why adult weight-loss programs are just not right for children. First and foremost, children are growing and healthy weight is a moving target that keeps changing. It is hard for parents to know if a child should be losing, maintaining, or gaining weight. Importantly, losing weight too quickly could prevent a child from growing properly. That is why this book encourages parents to work closely with a child's doctor to set the right healthy-weight goals for that child.

Moreover, children should not be on the structured type of diet that adults often follow. Structured diets are too restrictive and do not teach a child healthy eating habits for life. Instead, when children live a healthy lifestyle with the help of parents who follow the 5 Rules and 5 roles described in this book, the weight will take care of itself. On every page, *Family Power: 5 Simple Rules for a Healthy-Weight Home* tackles the challenge of healthy weight with useful, practical information. It distills the best of scientific literature and puts it into readable form that parents can use. The 5 Rules and 5 roles represent the consensus of world experts who work in this field. This book is a very powerful tool for parents to have in hand, whether they are trying to deal with weight challenges on their own or with help from their child's pediatrician or doctor.

So much of today's problem with children and weight is due to factors in society. None of us as individuals can change general societal trends like increased car time, greater use of remote control devices, televisions, and computers, and less activity in our daily lives. That is why this book is such a valuable tool. It will help parents make small changes in their own lives that will make a big difference to their children.

I have dedicated my career to the health of our children through my specialty practice as a pediatrician as well as through my work with the American Academy of Pediatrics Task Force on Obesity and Committee on Nutrition. Children are our future. With the rules and roles described in this book, we can help harness the power of the family today so that children can lead productive, happy, and, importantly, healthy lives throughout their childhood and well into their adult years.

—Marc S. Jacobson, M.D.

Acknowledgments

First, an enormous thank you to the families who participated in the Weight Watchers pilot program and the coaches who helped them in their efforts to establish, support, and sustain a healthy-weight home. Special thanks to those family members who shared their personal stories in this book. Their experiences and insights provide the reality behind the science and show that creating a healthy-weight home is indeed possible.

Besides the family portraits in part two, several families took the time to tell us about their experiences and to share the tips and strategies that were working well for them. While they are not mentioned by name, you will see their many contributions to this book. Thank you to the Clark, Driggs, Moore, Rivero, Williams, Ramer, Sherlock, Wiebe, Wiest, and Zajac families.

I am indebted to the researchers, physicians, and scientists who contributed to making the Family Power pilot program a reality, especially the pediatricians of the Pediatric Health Alliance in Tampa, Florida: Drs. Lane France, Rick Wilde, and Jackie Hartman. Thanks also to Dr. Michael Lowe for his valuable insights and guidance in shaping numerous chapters in this book.

Last but far from least, thanks to the Weight Watchers International team. *Family Power* would not have gotten started without the help of Linda Huett, Jonas Fajgenbaum, Cheryl Horning, Barbara Dutton

xii   ACKNOWLEDGMENTS

Weingarten, and Susan Learner Barr. This book would not have happened without the commitment and indefatigable efforts of Mindy Hermann and Evren Bilimer, as well as those of our editor, Tom Miller. Thank you.

Karen Miller-Kovach, M.S., R.D.

Introduction

by Meredith Vieira

I wish that books like *Family Power* had been around during my childhood years. When I was growing up, I was a chubby kid who was very self-conscious about weight. Families did not discuss or deal with weight issues in those days, so I handled my weight issues on my own—the wrong way. I tried lots of different strategies that just didn't work: fad diets, tossing food out the window, lying about eating. And worst of all, I grew into adulthood still being uncomfortable with my own body.

Once I started a family, my attitude toward dealing with weight issues changed. I wanted to prevent my children from experiencing the same weight and body image problems I had suffered. As a parent, I wanted to help my family find the right balance of health and happiness, and I realized that I needed to set an example for living a healthy lifestyle as well as to create one for my children. *Family Power* is filled with stories of and tips for how each of us can create a family environment where both nutrition and physical activity are things to enjoy. You're never too young or too old to learn!

One of the strengths of *Family Power* is that it presents extremely important research in a way that is easy for the reader to understand. I was particularly surprised to read that research has shown that when it comes to dieting and weight issues, children should not be treated as small adults—they have very different nutritional and caloric needs from grownups. This fact clearly calls for parents to use a much different strategy when helping children to achieve a healthy weight than they would use for themselves. I was also impressed to read in *Family Power* about how important it is for parents to understand that their children need calories to grow as well as the recommendation that most children should not lose more than one pound per month—advice very different from weight-loss recommendations for adults.

We recently dealt with a weight issue in my family. When my oldest son, Ben, was in eighth grade he gained weight, probably because his body was storing fuel prior to his growth spurt. Because my husband, Richard, and I had both been overweight at that age, we understood how important it was for us to help Ben without making him feel self-conscious. So the three of us became a team for healthy living: We all learned to read food labels so we could choose healthier foods to have at home. Our focus was on health—not on dieting or weight loss. Moderation became our buzzword, and we learned that we could enjoy treats and not feel denied. Ben was self-motivated because he wanted to try out for the high school soccer team. He took the lead, ate in a healthy way, increased his physical activity, and grew into his weight. I am very impressed that *Family Power* offers families many strategies for dealing with similar issues.

The *Family Power* chapters on physical activity are particularly important. The more active kids can be, the better. In our family, Richard and I are role models for physical activity. Both of us try to be active each day, either outdoors or at the gym. Richard is an inspiration for the kids—he has multiple sclerosis and yet is physically active every day. Ben and his brother, Gabe, are active in both structured school activities and in their leisure time spent with friends. Unfortunately for me, they no longer think that kicking a soccer ball with Mom is too much fun! Our daughter, Lily, enjoys dancing, and she and I also often take walks together.

One of the 5 Simple Rules in *Family Power* is to limit screen time.

In our home, we try to limit screen time to just the weekends. During the week the kids are so busy with school and activities that they have very little time to watch TV. Of course we make exceptions for special events like the World Series!

Kids with weight issues need to know that they're not in it alone. As *Family Power* eloquently shows, the family is a community that works together to live a healthier life.

PART ONE

What Is a Healthy-Weight Home?

As parents, we share the goal of providing the best possible lives for our children. Over the past few generations, however, providing the best possible life seems to come with a downside: excess weight. *Family Power: 5 Simple Rules for a Healthy-Weight Home* is about changing that. Its goal is to help our kids grow up to be lean and healthy adults. Excess weight gain in children is not limited to a certain age or gender; it can start anywhere from infancy to the late teen years. We must take steps to prevent our children from becoming overweight or to help them achieve a healthy weight if they are not at one now. It is never too late. By taking a close look at what scientists have found out about the weight management strategies that work for kids and combining them with the tips, strategies, and experiences of families that have been using them, *Family Power* shows you how to make a healthy-weight home.

What Is a Healthy-Weight Home?

A healthy-weight home is one in which everyone who lives there has a lifestyle that encourages them to be at a weight that is right and healthy for them. This means children and adults, including those who are very thin and those who are rather heavy. A healthy-weight home is not about being on a diet. It embraces meals and snacks that focus on wholesome, nutritious foods and it includes treats. Activity plays a vital role. Because parents create the home for their families, they are the "change agents" that make a healthy-weight home happen. This is done by surrounding the family with the 5 Simple Rules, using a style that will make them last.

You Are Not Alone

Over nine million American children over the age of six are the adult equivalent of obese. Over the past thirty years, the number of overweight two- to five-year-old kids in the United States has more than doubled. The number has more than tripled for children six to eleven years of age and for adolescents twelve to nineteen years of age over the same three decades. Researchers estimate that about 30% of children are either *at risk of overweight* or *overweight*.

The Institute of Medicine, a respected group that advises the government on health issues, describes childhood overweight as an epidemic. And while it often is not reported this way, experts agree that the solution lies in approaching the problem from every possible angle.

The problem of overweight children is not just a North American problem—it is happening all over the world. Researchers who looked at the rates of overweight in European thirteen-year-olds found the highest numbers in three very different countries: Finland, Ireland, and

Greece. Excess weight in children has even become an issue in countries where children never had problems, including China. A 2003 study conducted in Beijing, China, found that 28% of boys and 14% of girls were significantly overweight.

Experts agree that the main reason for this global trend lies in our kids' lifestyles—processed foods are replacing wholesome, less-processed foods; fast food is widely available; and the need to be active as part of daily life is declining. This lifestyle is nobody's fault. It is simply the course that our world has taken. Understanding the whys behind the trend is important, however, because it points us to the solutions. And when it comes to making a difference in the weight of our children, there are many strategies to take. How many and which ones depend on your lifestyle.

Making the Science Work for You

Childhood overweight is a complex issue. A number of factors are involved, from eating too many calorie-loaded foods to spending too much time in front of televisions, computer monitors, and video games. To add to the complexity, the definitions used to define excess weight in children are different from those for adults. We will explain this in chapter 1.

Several prestigious organizations, including the Institute of Medicine, the U.S. Surgeon General, and the American Heart Association, have reviewed the scientific studies on the development and treatment of childhood obesity and have issued recommendations. While valuable, these recommendations are generally meant to influence public policy, guide health care professionals, and create awareness about the issue. It is not always easy to translate the recommendations into "What can or should I be doing for my family?" That's why we've written this book.

Weight Watchers, as the largest provider of weight-loss services in the world, is concerned about the growing rate of overweight children and is committed to helping discover safe, lasting solutions. No one has more experience: since 1963, Weight Watchers has helped millions of people all over the world lose weight. With its science-based approach and talent for translating medical recommendations into practical advice that works in the real world, Weight Watchers is uniquely quali-fied to tackle this issue. This book provides you with the latest scientific information (a complete list of references is at the end of the book) that you can use to manage the weight and health of your entire family, including those who are underweight, overweight, or at a healthy weight now. But knowing and doing are two different things. *Family Power* goes beyond providing scientific information to bring you into the lives of the people who are taking the information and weaving it into their family's life.

The first part of the book lays the groundwork, providing the big pic-ture behind the 5 Simple Rules. It starts by taking a look at how excess weight is defined in children and how it is very different from over-weight in adults. Weight-loss recommendations for kids are also quite different from those for adults, so we include the current guidelines for children as well. One chapter looks at the science of changing behavior and how to increase the odds for success. This is followed by a chapter that explains the basics of weight management and why kids are not miniadults. The chapter shows that while the basic equation of calories in/calories out applies to everyone, changing the results of the equation are very much different for children. This leads into the 5 Simple Rules and the science that they come from. Finally, the roles that parents play in creating a healthy-weight home are defined. Throughout part one we include answers to the questions that parents often ask—everything from "Should I weigh my child?" to "What is the difference between a snack and a treat?"

With the background in place, part two goes into the whys and hows of making the Rules a part of family life. By focusing on each of the roles that all parents play—role model, provider, enforcer, protector, and advocate—the 5 Simple Rules are consistently reinforced. This is the magic that makes them work. The focus in part two is on the tips, strategies, and experiences of families who have taken on the task of weight management and are seeing success. Besides getting an in-depth look at many families who are using Family Power now, part two also has the advice of the coaches who have worked with these families and many, many more.

The book ends with some of the issues and challenges that many families may face as they work to create a healthy-weight home. From nontraditional family structures to having an unsupportive spouse, answers are given to often-asked questions on how to handle these situations, including how to get extra help if and when it is needed.

Kids Can Be More Successful Than Adults

When it comes to weight and children, there is good news. Kids have an *energy advantage* over adults. Unless they are older teens, kids are still growing and that takes energy (also known as calories). Children are also more responsive to being active than adults when they are given the opportunity. Because of this, children are likely to be able to achieve and sustain a healthy weight with fewer rules than most adults. In fact, living in a healthy-weight home—a home in which all family members live a lifestyle that supports nutritious eating and regular physical activity—can make a big difference in stopping and/or reversing the pattern of weight gain that leads to obesity. Making small, consistent changes in a few key areas rather than following a structured, low-calorie diet and strict exercise regimen is a realistic approach to both reducing excess weight in children and enhancing the health of all family members. *Family Power* shows you how.

The 5 Simple Rules

Rule #1:   Focus on wholesome, nutritious foods.

Rule #2:   Include treats.

Rule #3:   Aim to keep nonhomework screen time at two hours (or less) a day.

Rule #4:   Try to be active an hour or more a day.

Rule #5:   The Rules apply to everyone in the home.

EXPERT PORTRAITS

Family Power has been a team effort that includes weight-loss experts, pediatricians, coaches, and, most important, families. Throughout the book, we include portraits of some of the people who are behind *Family Power*. We hope that by getting to know them, you will feel comfortable and confident that following the 5 Simple Rules is right for your family.

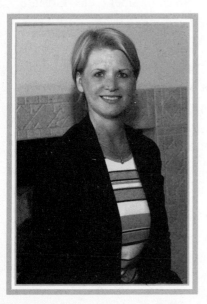

Karen Miller-Kovach, M.S., R.D.

As Chief Scientific Officer for Weight Watchers International, I am committed to helping those who want and need to lose weight. Weight Watchers has always taken a science-based approach to its programs and services. My job is to know the science and, if it does not exist, to help create the studies and trials that will give us the answers we need.

The Weight Watchers approach includes the four pillars that are known to provide lasting weight loss in adults:

1. Making wise food choices

2. Being physically active

3. Developing positive thinking skills

4. Living in a supportive environment

While the Weight Watchers approach has been developed and extensively studied in adults, it has not been rigorously evaluated in children. The fact is, none of the popular weight-loss methods have, so any recommendations about their use in children and adolescents are based on the assumption that what's right for adults is appropriate for kids.

Weight Watchers does not encourage children to join its program, and no child under the age of ten can become a member. For those between the ages of ten and seventeen, membership in our meetings-based program is available only with a doctor's referral, which is required to ensure that a health care professional who knows the child and the family has made an assessment and believes that the type of program that Weight Watchers provides is a good fit for that child. Access to the subscription weight-loss service on WeightWatchers.com is only available to adults.

Recognizing that popular adult-based programs had not been adapted and carefully studied in children and adolescents, Weight Watchers took on the challenge, resulting in the Family Power pilot project and this book. Since we were interested in exploring the impact parents have on the weight of their children, we developed a family-focused pilot program that called on parents to take the science-based recommendations that have been proven to affect children's weight and incorporate them into the eating and activity patterns of their homes. Rather than launch the pilot in a traditional clinical trial, we wanted to try it in the real world. In 2003, Weight Watchers joined forces with Pediatric Healthcare Alliance, a large pediatric group practice in Tampa, Florida, to pilot the family-focused approach. In 2005, the pilot was expanded to include the Orlando, Florida, and Seattle, Washington, areas, with more planned in the future. To learn more about the project, log on to www.weightwatchers.com/family.

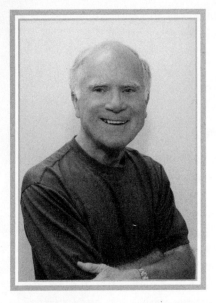

Lane France, M.D.

I am a pediatrician, heading a large group practice in Tampa, Florida, the Pediatric Healthcare Alliance. For years, I have been concerned about the problem of weight gain in children. I have seen many children in my career. Over the years, my patients have become heavier and heavier. I have made it a practice to talk with each and every parent and child about the importance of eating a nutritious diet and getting more physical activity.

I am passionate and persistent about this problem. Excess weight gain is one of the biggest problems in pediatrics today, and this is the first generation of children who may not live as long as their parents do. Reversing excess weight gain in our children is going to take a long time. Consider how much time it took to motivate people to take action to stop smoking, buckle up seat belts, and use helmets for bicycling and skating.

The saying goes: "It takes a village to raise a child." I feel that it indeed does take a village to tackle the growing problem of children who are too heavy. Weight gain in children is not the fault of parents, schools, pediatricians, or any one group, so it cannot be stopped through the actions of just one person or group. One day, I realized that my efforts might be more effective and reach more children if I involved the community.

Knowing that Weight Watchers shared my passion, we joined together. The Pediatric Healthcare Alliance patients were the first to learn about Family Power. Our doctors joined together to let parents know that they have the power to change their children's weight. Several (you'll meet two in chapter 13) joined the pilot program and spoke to the families you'll meet.

These are families just like yours. They come from all walks of life, but share the goal of helping their children to be as healthy as they can be. They are helping each other by creating a village of support to make a difference in their families' lives.

My goal is to work together with the movers and shakers of the community to help our children. I invited other pediatricians to collaborate with me and tell children and their parents about healthy weight. We formed a committee composed of a member of the school board, a reporter from our local paper, a nurse, several doctors, and a community leader to brainstorm ideas for getting the community involved. Since television has a big influence on parents and children, I am also talking with our local television personalities to get them on board.

The environment in all areas of the community has to change. Towns need trails, parks, and outdoor space for children to play in. I believe that schools should take treats out of the cafeteria and return physical education to the daily schedule. I also believe that parents have to turn off the television, the computer, and video games and promote exercise instead of sedentary activities. Family meals are essential. Let's work together to help children reach a healthy weight and to prevent children from gaining too much weight in the first place.

The problem is preventable as long as parents, schools, medical professionals, and leaders in the community recognize that something can be done if they work together. Kids and parents can't tackle the problem on their own. They need the help of the community, and every person helps.

Chapter 1

When Weight Is an Issue

The numbers don't lie. Children all around the world are gaining more weight faster than ever before. Despite this, there are good reasons to be optimistic. Several studies find that there are proven strategies that encourage kids to develop healthy eating and activity patterns that help them to stop gaining excess weight and let them "grow into" a healthy weight. Healthy-weight efforts that are directed toward kids are more

---

Some Definitions

BMI stands for Body Mass Index, a number that is used to evaluate body weight.

Overweight is the term used for children with a very high BMI for their age. Adults with a comparable BMI are defined as *obese*.

At risk of overweight is used for children whose BMI is between the healthy and overweight ranges. Adults with comparable BMIs are classified as *overweight*.

In this book, the terms *obese* and *obesity* are not used to refer to children who have a specific BMI, but rather to characterize the medical issues of excess weight in children and adults.

---

successful at keeping weight in the healthy range long term than they are with adults.

A Closer Look at BMI

Researchers around the world need technical definitions so that they can put studies into a common context. When it comes to weight, the definitions are based on a number called the Body Mass Index (BMI). BMI is used to evaluate body weight in both children and adults. For most people, BMI is a good indicator of the amount of fat on the body. BMI can be calculated by plugging one's body weight and height into the BMI formula, or it can be looked up on a chart. The BMI calculation is the same for everyone—men and women, adults and children. Adults can find out their BMI by checking the BMI chart on any of a number of government or health organization Web sites.

Web Sites for Determining Adult BMI

www.WeightWatchers.com

www.consumer.gov/weightloss/bmi.htm

www.nhlbi.nih.gov/guidelines/obesity/bmi_tbl.htm

www.shapeup.org

www.obesity.org

Weight-related categories for adults, namely, underweight, healthy weight, overweight, and obese, are determined by dividing BMIs into ranges. For adults, a BMI of 19 or lower is considered underweight, a BMI of 19 to 24.9 is a healthy weight, a BMI between 25 and 29.9 is overweight, and a BMI of 30 or more is obese. The categories and BMI cutoff points are the same for adult men and women of all ages.

The BMI calculation for children uses the same formula as for adults and is based on weight and height (or length for very young children). Charts called BMI-for-age charts are used to track a child's growth over time. BMI-for-age charts consider the child's age because BMIs change depending on a child's state of development. And because boys and girls grow and develop differently by age, separate BMI charts are used for boys and for girls.

Parents often ask . . .

Won't our pediatrician tell us if our child's weight is higher than the healthy range?

While this would be ideal and professional pediatric organizations are encouraging doctors to include this information as part of routine care, some pediatricians do not always share this information with you. It may be because they have their minds on something else or because they assume that you already know it. The bottom line is, if the doctor does not tell you your child's BMI-for-age, ask.

Pediatricians include the BMI-for-age chart in a child's medical record. At each routine visit, the pediatrician or nurse plots BMI-for-age on the growth chart and compares the result to standards for the child's age, as well as standards for growth over time.

BMI-for-age is not as simple as weight, but it is a more accurate way to evaluate a child's body weight. It corresponds well to levels of body fat—a high BMI-for-age usually means that a child has a lot of body fat. Pediatricians use BMI-for-age to follow a child's body size from childhood through adolescence and into adulthood.

Parents often ask . . .

How can I tell if my child is overweight or just big for his age?

It is very difficult simply to look at a child and tell if he or she is overweight. As kids grow and develop, their body shape changes. The only real way to know the difference between big and overweight is to plot the information on a BMI-for-age chart. Because this information is part of your child's medical record, a quick call to the doctor's office can tell you.

How BMI Changes as a Child Grows

The BMI-for-age chart helps pediatricians tell the difference between normal weight gain during growth and too much weight gain. Looks can be deceiving when it comes to weight in children, so health care professionals rely on the BMI-for-age chart to guide them. For example, it is not uncommon for infants and toddlers to look chubby but have a BMI in the healthy range.

BMI, body shape, and body size change throughout childhood. As a child moves from being a toddler to being a preschooler, BMI typically drops and growth slows to about 2.5 pounds of weight per inch of height growth. After the preschool years, BMI gradually increases. Going from the late elementary school years and into the very beginning of puberty, children's bodies can look very different from each other. Some kids grow much faster than others, and body shapes change. Some children gain body fat before they grow taller because their body is storing fat to prepare for the rapid growth spurt that goes with puberty.

During puberty, boy's and girl's bodies change in different ways.

A boy's body adds muscle and usually loses body fat, but boys develop more fat in their bellies. A girl's body adds both muscle and body fat, with fat going to her breasts, hips, and buttocks. Research shows that girls are more likely than boys to gain excess weight during adolescence.

Parents often ask . . .

One of my children is really thin. Does that mean she is anorexic?

Not necessarily. Anorexia nervosa, a medically diagnosed eating disorder, has several characteristics besides a low weight, including things like voluntary starvation, excess exercise, eating rituals, and an abnormal perception of body weight. If you have any concerns about your daughter, it's worth a trip to your family doctor (with a call before the visit to discuss your concerns) for an evaluation. If needed, your doctor will be able to refer you to other professionals for more help (we discuss this in chapter 15).

Why Children Are Not Obese

Strictly speaking, there are no obese children. Although people often use the terms "overweight" and "obese" when describing children with excess weight, "obese" does not apply to children. The U.S. Centers for Disease Control and Prevention (CDC) uses only "risk of overweight" or "overweight" for children and adolescents whose BMI-for-age is above the healthy-weight range.

It is not uncommon for people, including the media and many health professionals, to use the terms "overweight" and "obese" and not be referring to the technical definitions. Since BMI standards for "overweight" in children correspond closely with BMI standards for "obese"

GENERAL GUIDELINES FOR GENDER-SPECIFIC BMI CUTOFFS			
	Boys		Girls
Age	At Risk for Overweight If BMI Is Greater Than	Overweight If BMI Is Greater Than	At Risk for Overweight If BMI Is Greater Than	Overweight If BMI Is Greater Than
2 years	18.2	19.3	18.0	19.1
5 years	16.8	17.9	16.8	18.3
8 years	18.7	21.2	18.3	20.7
13 years	23.0	27.0	23.8	28.3
18 years	26.9	30.6	27.3	33.1

Source: www.cdc.gov/growthcharts/.

in adults, people often treat the two words as if they mean the same thing. This makes reading articles in newspapers, magazines, or even medical journals confusing, because it can be hard to figure out exactly which weight classifications are being referred to. Generally, if an information source refers to childhood obesity, it most likely means that the children were in the overweight category.

BMI Links between Childhood and Adulthood

Kids with a high BMI-for-age are more likely to become obese adults. The longer a child is overweight, the more likely it is that he or she will have adult weight issues. About 33% of preschool children with excess weight become obese adults. About 50% of school-age children will do so. In general, children with a high BMI are twice as likely to develop adult obesity as children whose BMI is in the healthy range. The risk is greatest for children who have the highest BMI and who maintain a high BMI at older ages.

Children who carry excess weight with them into adulthood are also more likely to have weight-related illnesses, including heart disease and diabetes. The bottom line is that preventing excess weight

Parents often ask . . .

If my child is already overweight, does that mean she will automatically become an obese adult?

While overweight children have a greater risk of taking their excess weight into adulthood, it is not true that they will necessarily become obese adults. In fact, half of school-age children who are overweight do not become obese adults. Children who are already overweight benefit by living in a healthy-weight home and either preventing more weight gain or reducing their weight.

gain at as early an age as possible is ideal. Bringing a high BMI down into the healthy range is also important. Beyond health issues, there are also avoidable social and financial consequences to being an overweight teen.

While sobering, these findings should not be discouraging. Children have a distinct advantage over adults when it comes to weight management. They need more calories as they grow, so it is simpler to make small changes in eating and activity patterns that can have a big impact on their body weight. Moreover, children who learn the principles of a healthy-weight lifestyle are likely to apply them to their adult lives, leaving them with the legacy of a healthy weight.

Weight-Loss Recommendations

Current recommendations for the treatment of overweight in children have two goals. The first is to make sure that the child grows and develops normally. The second is to help the child gradually reach a healthy weight. Experts in the field of childhood obesity developed their weight-related recommendations with these two goals in mind.

Experts agree that it is best to start early, with children as young as three years of age. One strategy for young children is to slow their rate of weight gain so that their BMI-for-age does not keep going up. For example, a goal for very young children (two to four years of age) whose BMI-for-age is near the top of the range might be to limit weight gain to less than two pounds for every inch of growth. The other often recommended strategy is to maintain the child's weight while the child grows. As the child gets taller, BMI-for-age drops into the healthy-weight range. This approach is often recommended for children who are four years of age or older and who do not have medical problems from their weight.

Weight loss usually is not recommended for children up to seven years of age. The exception is a child with a BMI in the overweight range who already has a weight-related medical condition like high blood pressure or high blood cholesterol.

The recommendations are similar for children older than seven years of age. The goal for children whose BMI-for-age puts them in the at risk of overweight range is to maintain a steady weight as they grow taller. Children who are older than seven years, have a medical complication due to their weight, and have a high BMI might be encouraged to lose weight.

Adult-based weight loss programs are not appropriate for children, except for older teens who have reached their adult height and have a BMI of at least 30.

Weight-loss recommendations should be based on the age of the child, the degree of overweight, and the presence of any weight-related medical problems. Even when weight loss is recommended, it should be done in a slow and gradual way. The current recommendation is that children should not lose more than an average of one pound per month unless they are under the direct supervision of a pediatrician with experience in weight management. Even under a doctor's supervision, experts recommend a slow and gradual weight loss.

		Weight-Related Health Complications	
WEIGHT-LOSS RECOMMENDATIONS SUMMARY			
Age	**Range of BMI-for-Age**		**Treatment**
Up to 7 years	At risk of overweight, overweight	No	Weight maintenance
Up to 7 years	Overweight	Yes	Consider weight loss
Older than 7 years	At risk of overweight	No	Weight maintenance
Older than 7 years	At risk of overweight, overweight	Yes	Weight loss
Late teen years	BMI of at least 30	Yes or no	Weight loss on adult program

Small weight changes can add up over the course of the year. For example, losing a pound per month becomes 12 pounds after a year. Add a couple inches of growth and it is likely that BMI-for-age will drop even more. Slow weight loss lets a child grow taller at a normal rate and helps maintain muscle mass. Gradual loss is achievable. In addition, the eating patterns that provide for slow weight loss are easier to sustain and fuel normal growth and development.

Parents often ask . . .

Why is the recommended rate of weight loss so much lower for kids than for adults?

For several reasons, there is a big difference between the one to two pounds per week recommendation for adults and the one pound per month for kids. First, the nutritional needs of children are higher and they need a fair amount of food and calories to make sure that those needs are met. In addition, the more slowly weight is lost, the more likely it will stay off. Finally, to lose weight at a more rapid pace, a child would have to make big changes in the calorie balance equation. This can only be done with a highly structured program, and this type of approach usually backfires with kids.

Parents often ask . . .

Should I weigh my child and, if so, how often?

It is generally not a good idea to weigh a child because it sends the message that weight is very important. Because children are weighed as a regular part of their medical care, it is better to limit the actual weighing to those visits. As a week-to-week indicator, the way clothes are fitting gives you a good idea of what is going on.

Chapter 2

Getting Ready for Change

While it may seem impossible to predict whether or not a person will be able to make a change in his or her behavior, whether it is to stop smoking or reduce credit card debt, there is actually a lot of science behind behavior change. Working through the change process as part of creating a healthy-weight home increases the likelihood for success.

Weight and Behavior Change

Many people think that weight loss is a behavior change. In fact, it is not. Body weight is actually the *result* of many, many behaviors that include both food and activity, everything from how many soft drinks are consumed to how many hours are spent watching television. If weight gain is a problem, the only way to stop it is to change some—but not necessarily all—of the behaviors that are behind the gain. If weight loss is a goal, either more behaviors need to be changed or more significant changes need to be made to a few behaviors.

Our lives are very busy. Often, the thought of making a big change—including working toward a healthy-weight home—can be overwhelming. The 5 Simple Rules may be simple, but they are not easy to tackle all at once because they involve so many parts of our everyday lives—everything from what we eat, to making time to exercise, to how we handle stress.

It is nearly impossible, and it is not recommended, to try to follow every one of the Rules at once. Instead, it works better to take small, progressive steps and make changes one at a time.

Most of us are ready to make some of the recommended changes but not others. That's okay. For example, you may feel comfortable adding an after-dinner walk as a family activity, but you may not be comfortable with cutting down on fast-food meals. Again, that's okay. Focusing first on those changes that are realistic is the smart way to go. It also improves the chances that the changes you do make will become part of the family's routine.

It is also not necessary to follow all the 5 Simple Rules completely. Because weight is determined by literally hundreds (or thousands) of small behaviors, we have the opportunity to pick and choose which strategies will be used and how closely they will be followed. Consistency in making a few changes is more likely to lead to lasting success than trying to do everything at once.

Parents often ask . . .

What if we are ready to change but our kids are not?

This is one of those times when being the adult in charge helps. Parents set the family policies and are in a position to make changes even when there is resistance from the kids. The trick is to pick changes that will meet the least resistance and then implement them in a realistic and consistent way. Over time, resistance usually decreases because the reality of the change is not as bad as anticipated. And when kids start to reap the benefits the changes bring, resistance to more changes is less likely.

Behavior change is an ongoing process. As parents, we can judge our families' success over time and, if it makes sense, add more changes to push things along. We can also see if we've gone too far and pull back on the changes if that makes sense. Forcing changes a family is not ready, willing, or able to make is unhelpful because the changes are likely to be met with a lot of resistance. That means they are not likely to last very long.

The Science of Change

Two pioneers in the field of changing behavior, James Prochaska and Carlo DiClemente, identified *stages of change* to help people evaluate how ready they are to make a change in their behavior. This framework of change stages can help a family to decide what behaviors or steps toward a healthy-weight home they can reasonably make.

The first stage, *precontemplation*, means that change is not even on the family's radar screen. For example, if it is the family's habit to have soft drinks with meals, the idea of switching to water or low-fat milk has never even been considered. The goal of precontemplation is to get a behavior on the radar screen. Learning about the 5 Simple Rules and the science behind them is a good first step to creating awareness about the behaviors that make a healthy-weight home. After this is done, the decision as to what specific behaviors a family wants to work on begins.

In the second stage, *contemplation*, some thought is being given to making a general change—for example, including more family activities, but a specific plan or time period to make it happen does not exist. This is the time to think about the various behaviors that make up a healthy-weight home and decide which ones are worth taking to the next step.

Preparation, the third stage, involves looking into the specific ways to actually make the change. It means planning for the change and picking a date to make it happen. For example, let's say that switching from soft drinks to low-fat milk at meals is a behavior change the family is going to make. To prepare for the change, it is likely that more milk will be needed and the number of soft drinks kept in the house can be reduced. If there is already a lot of soda pop in the house, a week or two to use it up may be allotted. Then, on the next trip to the grocery store, the new amounts of milk and soft drinks are bought. This sets the stage for a successful implementation of the change, and the target start for the change can be the meal following the shopping trip.

It is during the preparation stage that decisions about what strategies to use to make a change happen take place. Besides a plan and a start date, preparation often means getting information. For example, if a goal is to find new activities that a family will enjoy, exploring the classes offered at the local Y, reading community bulletins, or checking out local parks can help give specific choices about how to make the change a reality.

In the change process, the preparation stage tends to be relatively short. Enough time needs to be given to work out an achievable plan, but it is generally recommended that the projected start date be within the next month. If start dates repeatedly come and go without the plan being acted on, it is a sign that the change is really in the contemplation phase and some rethinking is in order.

In the *action* phase, the plans made during the preparation phase are put into place. During this time the change is new, so it may take some getting used to. Sticking to the plan for at least several days is recommended at this point. Motivation is often high, which increases the chances for success. It is not uncommon, however, for the plans that were made during preparation to require some modification. That is okay. It is much easier to make some adjustments to a good plan to make it fit better into a family's life than to try to stick with a plan that is not working. If it is not working, it is unlikely to last.

The *maintenance* phase marks the time when the change has made its way into becoming a part of a family's everyday life and routines. The change is now simply the way things are done, and to make it different at this point would require another change. That said, change is a part of life, and periodic adjustments will need to be made even during maintenance. For example, if the family's habit is to walk after dinner and one of the kids takes on another activity during this time, an alternative time or a different activity may be needed.

Before trying to create a healthy-weight home, it is helpful to get a sense of a family's readiness to make specific changes in eating and activity patterns. This includes adults and children alike. The time spent going through this exercise is very helpful because a lack of readiness to change is often not as important as why an adult or a child is not ready to change.

For example, a child may say that she is not ready to have only a couple of treats a day. When asked why, she may say that she is afraid of being hungry. By understanding that fear, it may make sense to let that change go for now and instead focus on providing more wholesome, nutritious foods. Because these foods are so filling, the child may have less hunger and then be ready to eat fewer treats.

Parents often ask . . .

What if I'm ready but my spouse is not?

Forcing change on anyone, whether it is an adult or a child, is unlikely to work. In many ways, it is harder for adults to change because they have had more years learning and getting comfortable with the habits they have. Rather than trying to force the change, it is better to understand the whys behind the resistance.

If the change is not important to your spouse, helping your spouse understand the benefits for the children of making the change may help. If it is a matter of confidence (and many adults lack confidence that they can change their habits), then promising encouragement and support in making the change is the way to go.

Importance and Confidence

There are two additional things to consider when looking at readiness to change. The willingness to make a change is directly connected to a person's feelings about whether the change is worthwhile (its importance) and whether it is achievable (confidence that it can happen). When it comes to many behaviors that make up eating and activity, the importance and confidence feelings are not always obvious. For example, a teenager may say that he is not ready to be more active. In discussing the why behind the lack of readiness, it may be that the young man knows how important activity is to weight management but lacks confidence in his physical abilities. By finding some activities he will enjoy and that do not require a lot of skill, as well as bolstering his confidence with words of encouragement (and maybe doing the activity along with him), a parent can build a teen's confidence. With more confidence, he will be more likely to include activity in his day.

Parents often ask . . .

How do I balance my priorities as a parent?

This is a tough question and one that parents need to figure out on their own. What is essential, however, is to be realistic and not expect too much of yourself. We all have more priorities than we can achieve, so choices need to be made. Often doing a little is better than doing nothing. But how much you can do while balancing all the challenges that make up being a parent can only be answered by you.

Readiness to create a healthy-weight home is not simply a matter of thinking it is important. The importance of taking on any new behavior has to be stacked up against all the other things that are important to a family. Indeed, behavior change happens only if the importance of following all or parts of the 5 Simple Rules takes priority over other important family matters.

Parents often ask . . .

How can I help my kids accept the importance of the 5 Simple Rules?

Children with weight issues usually want to lose weight but do not necessarily know how. Talking with kids about how the 5 Simple Rules will make a difference in their weight raises the importance because it changes things from a desire into a real possibility. Talking about the benefits a child is likely to get, including more energy and better-fitting clothes, also boosts the importance rating.

To make realistic decisions about what and how many changes can be made in creating a healthy-weight home, it helps to compare the expected benefits from making the change against the amount of time and effort it will take to make it happen. Picking those changes where the pros clearly outweigh the cons is the recommended way to go, especially at the beginning.

Creating Change through Goals

Successful behavior change has four necessary elements:

1. A specific, measurable goal that is realistically achievable

2. A plan to achieve the goal—what needs to happen

3. Believing that the goal is important

4. Having confidence that the plan can and will be implemented

Taking a Realistic Look at Behavior Change

- How badly is the change wanted?
- Will it make a difference in daily life?
- What are the benefits of the change?
- Why should behavior be changed?
- Is the change worth the time and effort?
- What changes will it make in the day's routines?
- What will the costs be in money, time, and effort?
- What are the good things about not changing?
- What would it be like to make the changes?
- What would need to happen to make it a higher priority than it is now?

In thinking about making a food or activity behavior change, the first question to ask is: "What would I like to happen?"—that is, naming the goal or actions. Goals can be small and simple as long as they are achievable and measurable.

Parents often ask . . .

Should everyone in the family have the same goals?

While the big goals should be shared by all family members, there may be different action steps. This is particularly true if there are older kids in the house. For example, family-based activities may not be realistic, so activities with friends or on a teen's own may make sense. But the larger goal of being active is everyone's goal.

Sample Goals

Increase family dinners from two to four nights per week.

Reduce playing video games from two hours per day to one hour per day.

Change from white rice and pasta to brown rice and whole-grain pasta.

Switch meal beverages from soft drinks or fruit juices to water or nonfat milk.

The second step is to ask: "What needs to happen for the goal to be met?" For example, if the goal is to have more family dinners, the action steps might include shopping and cooking over the weekend to save time, letting all family members know that they are expected to be at home for dinner on the designated days, and involving all family members in setting the table and serving the foods.

Evaluating how important a goal is and whether it can be accomplished may require a family discussion. When a family is working on a common goal and everyone has agreed to it, the goal is much easier to achieve. To make the goal a reality, each family member can take responsibility for parts of the action steps—a parent can cook and freeze the weekday dinners on the weekend, a younger child can set the table, and a teen can put the dinner in the oven when he or she gets home from school.

Finally, parents and family members need to take a look at the goal, the action steps, and who is going to do what to make it happen. When all these steps are in place, it usually becomes very clear whether or not a goal is likely to actually happen.

Chapter 3

Kids Are Not Little Adults

Whether a person is an adult or a child, if his or her body weight is the result of hundreds or thousands of food and activity behaviors, wouldn't it make sense that the weight-loss strategies that work in adults would be good for children too? For years, that's what many experts assumed, and a lot of people still subscribe to this point of view. However, that line of thinking is changing. That is one reason why the weight-loss recommendations for children are so different from those for adults and why the American Dietetic Association has different certification programs for dietitians treating adults and those treating kids.

Parents often ask . . .

Why don't adult weight-loss programs work for most kids?

It is believed that the main reason kids do not do well in programs designed for adults is that adult programs have too much structure and not enough family support. Kids do not generally need the type and amount of structure that adults need to manage their weight. Asking kids to follow a strict diet and/or exercise regime can cause them to resist and create conflicts at home. A strict regime is often abandoned to avoid the conflicts that it brings. To overcome this resistance, a family-based approach that is not overly strict and is done with a lot of support makes more sense.

When adult weight-loss treatments have been used in kids, the results have been disappointing, and strict diets have even been linked with some pretty scary consequences like eating disorders. While kids and adults share a lot of physical traits, there are also some sizeable differences.

It's All about Energy Balance

One similarity that adults and children have is the law of thermodynamics, because it works the same for everyone. This law says that how much any person weighs is ultimately the result of calories in and calories out. Put another way, it is a result of the calories that we eat in the form of food and beverages and the calories that we burn to meet our body's need for energy and, for children, growth.

A child whose BMI-for-age remains in the same percentile year after year is balancing the number of calories eaten with the calories needed to grow and develop. If a child is gaining weight at a rate faster than needed for growth, it means that the calories in are greater than the calories out. The result will be a progressive increase in the BMI-for-age. Conversely, a decrease in the BMI-for-age can only happen if weight is lost or weight gain is less than the calories needed to account for what is needed for growth. Sometimes this is referred to as growing into the weight.

Parents often ask . . .

How many calories does my child need?

While this may seem like an easy question, it is not. Trying to estimate the caloric needs of a child is like trying to hit a moving target. Kids grow in fits and spurts, and their energy needs go right along with that. Also, the number of calories they burn in activity varies tremendously from day to day. Rather than trying to figure out a number of calories, a better strategy is to pay attention to food choices and let children's hunger and fullness cues lead the way.

Changes to either side of the calorie equation can lead to a lower BMI-for-age. In a healthy-weight home, the calories-in side of the equation is reduced by focusing on foods and beverages that are lower in calories and higher in nutrients. These are also known as low-energy density, high-nutrient density foods because they pack a lot of nutrition into a single serving and the number of calories per serving tends to be low.

The calories-out side of the equation has two different elements. The first is physical activity, which burns calories. The second is time spent in sedentary activities that do not burn many calories, like television watching or playing video games. These two elements are closely linked, because reducing the amount of time spent being sedentary frees up time for activity.

Parents often ask . . .

Is my child overweight because he eats too much or because he doesn't get enough exercise?

While there are occasional situations where clearly one or the other is the major reason for a calorie imbalance, for most kids the answer is a bit of both. This means that strategies to reduce weight gain need to pay attention to both food and activity.

Genes

One of the things that make all biological families a family is a common gene pool. There is no question that the risk of gaining excess weight is higher in families in which obesity is common. But we also know that genes are not behind the weight gain that many of our children are experiencing today. Genetic changes take generations and generations to show up; they cannot develop over the course of a few decades.

Parents often ask . . .

Why do some of my kids have weight issues and others do not?

There is no one answer. While biological families share a common gene pool, each person has a different mix. This means that some children might be more vulnerable to weight gain than others. It also means that the vulnerability may not be seen until a child is older. Also, every child has a unique personality, and these personal traits can have a big effect on weight-related behaviors.

Moreover, there is a big difference between having an increased risk for becoming overweight and actually becoming overweight. Biology is not destiny, and several studies find that it is not uncommon for overweight children to become adults with a healthy weight. In one study, 31% of obese children went on to become lean adults. Likewise, however, being a thin child does not protect against becoming overweight as an adult. In the same study, about another 30% of children who were lean grew up to develop obesity as adults.

A family-based approach like the one in *Family Power* has been shown to have lasting results on the entire family. In one study that looked at the weight change of all the family members who participated in a family-based program, the parents' change in BMI predicted the change in BMI-for-age for their children. This suggests that sharing a gene pool and living in a healthy-weight home helps everyone.

The Biggest Factor: Time

Another factor that adults and children share is a lack of time. Changing behaviors takes time. In one family-based weight program, families said that a lack of time was the biggest reason for not following the eating and activity recommendations. Time is a major issue for adolescents. Researchers looking at a group that included urban teenage girls found that the girls who were not active said that it was because they didn't have enough time. In the same study, however, those girls who wanted to lose weight, believed in the importance of exercise, were active with friends, or participated in a team sport were most likely to be active.

The reality is that no one can create more time, but making progress toward a healthy-weight home can be achieved within the twenty-four-hour day that we all have. It is a matter of carefully picking the changes to be made and being consistent in applying them so that they make it to the maintenance phase of the stages of change without taking a lot of time.

How Kids Are Different

Although weight is all about calories in and calories out, the equation doesn't work the same way for kids that it does for adults. Children, unlike adults, also need additional calories for growth and development. Children who eat about the number of calories that they need for growth, daily metabolism, and physical activity gain weight at a pace that is in line with their growing height. Children who eat more calories than they need gain weight beyond what is needed to support their added inches; those who eat less become thinner in relation to their growing height. If a child has a severe shortage of calories, his or her growth in height may slow down.

Both adults and children with weight issues are eating more calories than their body needs, but kids' typical diets are different from those of adults. In the United States, the typical child's diet is high in fat, the nutrient that is the most concentrated in calories—each teaspoon of fat contains about 40 to 45 calories (each teaspoon of pure protein or carbohydrate has about 20 calories). Chips, hot dogs, fried chicken, french fries, and cookies are just a few of the high-fat foods in a typical child's diet. Most kids also get extra calories from foods that provide a lot of calories in relation to their nutritional value, including fruit juices, soft drinks, and snack foods.

The activity patterns of adults and children are also different, and this affects body weight. Adults tend to be more sedentary because they have jobs that do not require much movement. Children today are typically less active than the kids of previous generations. This lack of activity is closely linked with increased screen time—more time spent watching television, working and playing on the computer, or playing video games. Lack of physical activity means that even if today's children were not eating more calories (which they are), their weight would still be increasing because they are spending fewer calories on activity. It is the double whammy of more calories in and fewer calories out that is causing the gains in kids' body weights to happen so quickly.

While different food and activity choices may be making children and adults gain weight, these choices are not the biggest difference between kids and adults. That difference is home life.

Adults live independently and are pretty free to make their own choices. Kids are not. One of the greatest advances in understanding childhood weight loss has to do with studies that look at the influence that parents have on their children's behavior. When it comes to weight loss, there is a direct link between adults and their behaviors. In children, the behaviors are mediated through the family, and this affects how and why a child will change.

Parents often ask . . .

If my child has a weight problem and I don't, why do I have to change?

You need to change because, as a parent, you are the biggest influence on your child's life. Making the changes with your child shows support and family solidarity. When it comes to kids and weight, that makes all the difference. In addition, you'll improve your health too.

Research shows that children rely on their parents to create behavior change. When they are young, the dependence is complete. As the child grows, the relationship evolves from parents making almost all the decisions to parents teaching the child how to create change for him- or herself. This includes how to evaluate readiness for change, set goals, make action plans, and follow through. Studies also find that parenting style makes a difference, as does a child's support system. For children, their primary support network is their family.

When it comes to weight loss, kids are a lot more complicated than adults. Still, they are also more likely to achieve weight-loss success when the approach used with them is based on sound science and when a wide range of behavior techniques are used. By expanding the ways that the basics of a healthy-weight home are put into action—for example, being a role model, providing wholesome foods, and enforcing rules consistently—it is possible to shape children's choices.

Parents often ask . . .

What should I do if my child starts talking a lot about weight?

The best approach is to try to shift the thinking from weight to being healthy. Weight management is, after all, about healthy living. By talking about the 5 Simple Rules and how they help achieve a healthy body weight, the focus is put on how to make positive changes and away from a number on a scale.

Chapter 4

The 5 Simple Rules

Weight management is about balancing the calorie equation. When it comes to calories in—food—two factors come into play: focusing on eating a lot of low-calorie, high-nutrition foods and reducing the number of high-calorie, low-nutrition foods. The calories out—activity—side of the equation also has two factors: being physically active and reducing sedentary time. These four factors are the foundation for the first four of the 5 Simple Rules. The fifth rule holds the key to the power that families have to create a healthy-weight home.

Rule #1: Focus on wholesome, nutritious foods.

A healthy-weight diet is one that emphasizes wholesome, nutritious foods. Most of these foods are high in vitamins, minerals, and other important nutrients and low in calories. These foods become the mainstay of a family's diet and are prominent in every meal and snack. Focusing on wholesome, nutritious foods not only enhances the achievement of a healthy weight, it also promotes overall health and well-being.

Parents often ask . . .

How can this approach work without counting calories?

When we look at the extra calories kids eat, they are not usually coming from wholesome, nutritious foods. They are coming from treats. By eating more wholesome foods and fewer treats, calories are automatically reduced. And because wholesome foods are also more filling, less total food is eaten and calories are further reduced. In contrast, cutting calories without paying attention to food choices can leave your child hungry.

Choose whole grains whenever possible. Foods made with whole grains like whole wheat or oats contain the nutrition benefit of all parts of the grain kernel. Whole-grain foods—100% whole wheat bread, brown rice, whole wheat pasta, and whole-grain cereal—also contribute fiber, a nutrient that helps keep the intestine healthy and boosts feelings of fullness. A diet rich in dietary fiber is recommended for children and adults. Indeed, a higher fiber diet can reduce problems with constipation, a common ailment in kids.

Making the switch from refined grains to whole grains is usually an easy adjustment, especially for kids, because it involves a one-to-one exchange of one food for another. Examples include substituting brown rice for white rice, corn tortillas for flour tortillas, and 100% whole wheat bread for white bread, and switching to whole-grain breakfast cereals and whole wheat pasta.

Make water, other noncaloric beverages, and low-fat or nonfat milk the household drinks of choice. Drinking calorie-containing soft drinks is an everyday part of many kids' lives. Between 1977 and 1994, soft drink consumption increased 41% in the United States. At the same time, milk intake dropped. This trend has been frequently linked with weight gain. Experts find that total calories go up as the amount of soft drinks goes up and that reversing the soft drinks trend makes a difference. One study in the United Kingdom found that those children who simply cut back on soft drinks lost weight over the course of a year, while the children who did not cut back gained weight. Fruit juices, while having nutritional value, also pack a lot of calories if they are used as a means to quench thirst. For this reason, the American Academy of Pediatrics (AAP) recommends that the total intake of calorie-containing nonmilk beverages, including 100% fruit juice, be limited to half a cup per day.

Parents often ask . . .

Shouldn't kids drink whole milk and aren't 100% fruit juices healthy?

The American Heart Association recommends whole milk for the first two years, followed by a switch to low-fat or nonfat milk and dairy products. Kids over the age of two do not need the calories or saturated fat that comes with full-fat milk. Regarding 100% fruit juice, it is healthy if you are only looking at providing some vitamins and minerals. When it comes to weight, it is not helpful because it provides a lot of calories without giving a feeling of fullness. Kids are better off getting their vitamins and minerals from food and not from a juice, except as a treat.

Include lots of fruits and vegetables a day. Fruits and vegetables supply nutrients and other healthful compounds that no other foods can supply. They also have a high content of both water and fiber, contributing to a feeling of fullness without supplying a lot of calories. Filling up on vegetables is an especially useful strategy to help children eat fewer calories. In one study on children aged nine to fourteen, boys who ate the most vegetables had the biggest drop in BMI. Experts recommend that everyone strive to eat at least five servings of fruits and vegetables a day, with an appropriate portion size based on the age of the person. As a rule of thumb, an appropriate serving size is one tablespoon of fruit or vegetable for each year of a toddler's or preschooler's age. Over time, serving sizes will increase. To learn more about the recommended serving sizes for various age groups, log on to the My Pyramid Web site (www.mypyramid.gov).

Parents often ask . . .

I have heard that diets cause eating disorders. Will following the 5 Simple Rules trigger an eating disorder in my child?

No. The 5 Simple Rules and parenting roles that make up Family Power can help kids avoid the emotional triggers that spark eating disorders. Having a healthy-weight home is all about eating well and being active without a lot of pressures about body weight, shape, or size.

Take in small amounts of healthy oils. While eating less fat is an effective way to eat fewer calories, it also can reduce the intake of vitamin E, an essential nutrient that is found in certain oils. Including small amounts of oils like canola oil or olive oil helps everyone, children and adults alike, to get the vitamin E that they need. Using small amounts of salad dressing and sautéing meats and vegetables in canola or olive oil are two easy strategies for adding these oils to the diet.

Be on the lookout for hidden fats and sugars in purchased and prepared foods. Most packaged and prepared foods include fats or sugars that increase calories without increasing nutrition. Many of us have come to rely on these foods because they taste good and are convenient. However, preparing simple, wholesome meals from basic foods like lean meats, fresh produce, and whole grains can take very little time and be just as tasty. Look for quick and simple ways to prepare meals, including baking, grilling, sautéing, poaching, and steaming.

Always eat breakfast. Breakfast is the ideal time to get a start on the day by eating a whole-grain bread or cereal, fresh fruit, and calcium-rich milk. Eating a wholesome breakfast also offers healthy-weight benefits and eating the meal together as a family, if possible, fosters togetherness. Research finds that children who eat breakfast tend to be less overweight than children who don't. Making breakfast a regular part of the day is a good health habit that children will carry to adulthood. This is a big plus, because eating breakfast is also linked with maintenance of weight loss in adults.

Strive for regular meal and snack times whenever possible. Eating breakfast and having family dinners both offer numerous weight benefits. In contrast, children who snack frequently are likely to eat too many treats.

Have family meals as much as possible. Children who eat dinner at home with their family have a more nutritious diet than those who don't, because they learn from these meals how to enjoy a variety of foods and how to try new foods, and they become familiar with healthy-weight eating skills.

Studies indicate that family meals tend to be more balanced nutritionally than meals that are eaten out. Children who eat meals at home tend to eat more fruits, vegetables, and high-fiber foods. That's important because these foods are filling without having a lot of calories. Children who have their meals at home also drink fewer soft drinks and eat less fried food.

According to government figures, there was a nearly 300% increase in the amount of food that children ate away from home between 1977 and 1996. Fast-food restaurants are particularly popular among children. Children who eat fast food frequently are likely to consume more fat, carbohydrates, added sugars, and sugar-sweetened drinks, as well as less milk and fewer fiber-rich foods, fruits, and vegetables (except potato) than those who don't.

Rule #2: Include treats.

Treats are foods that generally pack a lot of calories, are low in nutritional value, and rate highly on providing feelings of pleasure. Examples of treats include soft drinks, most desserts, candy, and highly processed packaged foods.

Parents often ask . . .

What exactly is a treat?

There is not a specific list that puts foods into "wholesome" and "treat" columns. That is something that you have to decide based on your family's eating habits and readiness to change. However, a general rule is that if a food is highly processed, like a box of macaroni and cheese, contains a lot of sugar or fat, like ice cream, or is not making a nutritional contribution to the diet, like fruit snacks, it should be used as a treat.

Treats are an important part of life today. Including one or two daily treats, in reasonable portions, adds enjoyment to eating, reduces feelings of deprivation, and supports a realistic, sustainable eating pattern. An important phrase in the last sentence is *reasonable portions*, because just as our weight has grown over the past thirty years, so have the portion sizes of the foods we eat. The food portions typically served in restaurants, fast-food chains, and other places are up to eight times bigger than is recommended. This is a particular concern for us as parents, because it means that our children have never lived in a world of smaller portions, so they are completely unaware of what a recommended portion size is. To them, a 20-ounce bottle of a soft drink and a king-size candy bar are normal. Several studies find that kids tend to eat more when they are served larger portions.

Treats can and should be a routine part of daily life. It is never a good idea to use treats as a reward or to take them away as a punishment. Research shows that rewarding or punishing with treats makes them more desirable to kids. Living in a healthy-weight home teaches children that treats are a special but regular part of eating.

The exact definition of what constitutes a treat is very individual. Food likes and dislikes are personal and are shaped by age, personality, mood, genetics, and other factors. For this reason, decisions about what to eat as a treat food should be left to each family member. For example, you could choose to have a glass of wine with dinner, while your preschooler may prefer a fruit roll-up.

A treat is different from a snack. Children need snacks because their stomachs are too small to hold enough food just at meals. A snack is a minimeal—it focuses on wholesome, nutritious foods.

Rule #3: Aim to keep nonhomework screen time at two hours (or less) per day.

Computers, DVDs, video games, and television play a prominent role in the lives of the modern child. It is estimated that over 25% of school-age children watch at least four hours of television daily, and the daily number of hours in front of the television has been repeatedly linked to weight gain. In addition, research is sending an early-warning signal, finding that the childhood television-watching habits of the last generation are having weight-related consequences as those kids are becoming young adults. One study finds that adults who watched the most television as children weighed more and were less fit than those adults who watched less television as children.

Screen time directly affects weight because it takes a lot fewer calories to sit in front of a screen than it does to play outside. Providing easy access to screens, such as having televisions, computers, or video game systems in a child's room, is not helpful. Research finds that children who have a television in their bedroom are more likely to develop weight issues, probably because watching the television is so convenient.

Parents often ask . . .

Is it okay if I pull the televisions out of my kids' bedrooms but leave the one in my room?

If you read ahead to Rule #5, you'll see that the rules apply to everyone. Being a positive role model is probably the most important thing you can do, and keeping your TV goes in the opposite direction. If this is a change that you are not willing or able to make yourself, then you shouldn't ask your kids to do it either.

The AAP recommends limiting screen time for children older than two years of age to a maximum of two hours per day as a strategy to prevent overweight in children. (The AAP also recommends no screen time for children under the age of two.) In today's world of televisions and computers, this rule may seem unrealistic, unattainable, and even unreasonable. As a first step, families can evaluate how much time each member spends in front of screens. Small goals to reduce that time, with specific plans to use the time for another activity, can help. If possible, it also helps to keep television, video games, and computers out of bedrooms. A key benefit of limiting screen time is that doing so frees up time for spontaneous exercise and family-centered activities.

Rule #4: Try to be active an hour or more per day.

The 2005 Dietary Guidelines for Americans recommend that children get an hour of daily physical activity. That is the same amount recommended for adults who want to maintain a weight loss. Most kids currently get about thirty minutes of activity a day, or about half of what they should. Experts agree that the current level of activity is not enough to prevent excess weight gain or lead to weight loss in children.

While an hour a day may sound like a lot, it helps to understand that the recommendation includes all kinds of activity, both structured and unstructured—that means everything from playing outside after school to riding a bike to the store.

One useful strategy for many families is to have after-school playtime. A mother whom you'll meet in part two designated the hour after school as a no-homework and no-television time as a way to entice her children to be more active. She found that not only did they become more active, they were better able to concentrate on their homework after taking this break. If the kids are in after-school care, caregivers can be asked to implement this strategy.

Parents often ask . . .

If my child plays a sport or takes lessons of some kind (e.g., tennis, swimming, or dance), isn't that enough?

Probably not. Most sports teams and lessons involve only a few hours a week, falling short of the hour a day recommendation. To have a better idea, you can keep track of how much time is spent in the activity (and that means actually doing the activity and not standing around) for a week or two and then see how much, if any, additional activity is needed.

Schools cannot be relied on to make sure kids get the activity they need. Many schools have cut back on recess and physical education classes so that more time can be spent on academic subjects. Government reports show that in the 1990s, participation in gym classes dropped because physical education was no longer required in many schools. As a child ages, the amount of time spent in active play is likely to go down, and this is particularly true for those with weight issues. Regardless of weight, the opportunities are often limited for older children. Sports teams become more competitive and involve fewer athletes as kids progress through the school system. Many schools do not offer options for activity except for their organized sports teams.

Active time can take the place of sedentary time and is a lot of fun for families who play together. A child's wishes about what activities to include should be taken into consideration. While it is a common belief that signing a child up for a team sport is always a good idea, many kids prefer to be active in other ways, and this needs to be respected. What is done to meet the activity recommendation is not nearly as important as whether the child enjoys it. One study found that dancing and walking were particularly effective for increasing activity, decreasing inactivity, and lowering BMI in children.

Rule #5: The Rules apply to everyone in the home.

A healthy-weight lifestyle is not just for the children in the household or those family members who have weight issues. The Rules work best if everyone in the family follows them. All family members, including those who are at a healthy weight and those who are not, benefit from the better health practices that the Rules provide. Members of families with a history of excess weight benefit even more.

In today's world, it is not just family members who care for our kids. If both parents work, meals and snacks are often provided by others. Left on their own, caregivers may not know or understand how to prepare meals and snacks that focus on wholesome foods. Likewise, caregivers may not understand the importance of getting kids active. In creating a healthy-weight home, the rules need to apply to everyone, including caregivers. This can be done by providing specific instructions about meals and snacks, treats, screen time, and exercise. Making sure that the instructions are followed is important, because providing kids with consistent expectations is what makes the rules stick.

Chapter 5

The Roles Parents Play

Parents are like the sun in the center of a solar system, and their kids are the planets that orbit around it. Just as the sun's influence on its planets is enormous, so, too, is the effect that parents have on their children. Nowhere is this more obvious than in the impact that parents have on their children's food and activity habits. According to the American Academy of Pediatrics, kids' health is deeply affected by their parents' health, relationships, and parenting styles. It is we parents who are at the center of creating a healthy-weight home by making the 5 Simple Rules a part of family life.

The research on the role that we parents play in making a healthy-weight home has been going on for over thirty years. In the 1970s, research focused on children's weight issues as a part of particular family characteristics like the communication style (the way people spoke to each other, the support within the family and parental consistency), family life skills (parenting styles, the way decisions were made), and individual feelings (self-image). The general finding from this research was that the kids who were the most successful in managing their weight came from supportive families with good relations among the family members. In addition, the parents of the more successful kids used strategies and techniques that created a sense of responsibility and a positive self-image in their children.

> **Parents often ask . . .**
>
> **How much of a difference do I really make?**
>
> Probably more than you will ever know. From the moment of birth, our kids look to us for everything. Every habit that we have, from hating brussels sprouts to fidgeting, is something that influences our children. This does not mean that we need to be paranoid about the way we behave. It simply means that we make a big difference and that the little changes we make, regardless of the age of our kids, will have an influence.

As parents, we play five major roles as we go about making a healthy-weight home. We parents are *role models* who show our kids how to eat well and be active by doing it ourselves. We parents are *providers*, because we buy the foods that our family eats and the toys and sports equipment that encourage activity. We parents are also *enforcers* by setting our family's food and activity policies and then making sure they are consistently followed. As *protectors*, we parents look out for our kids. We are also *advocates*, extending our commitment outside the home.

Because we parents are the ones who make a healthy-weight home happen, it is important to really understand each of the five roles and how each works with the 5 Simple Rules. This chapter provides the basics about the roles that parents play. Part two takes the roles and breaks them down, going into detail, with real-life examples of families, just like yours, that are making the 5 Simple Rules work for them.

> **Parental Roles That Affect Children's Weight**
>
> Role model
>
> Provider
>
> Enforcer
>
> Protector
>
> Advocate

Parents often ask...

Is one role more important than the others?

While they are all important, the roles of role model, provider, and enforcer are most closely linked with weight. If it came down to the most important role, the winner would be role model. That does not mean that the others are not important, but without a role model, the likelihood of real change is reduced.

Role Modeling

According to the *American Heritage Dictionary*, a role model is someone who acts as a model in a behavioral way or in a social role with the intention that another person will imitate the behavior or role. It is sometimes said that every child needs a role model. As parents, we are the most significant role models our children will ever have. We are not the only ones, however. Research shows that in families with more than one child, older siblings are role models, and caregivers take on the role as well. This is one of the reasons why it is so important for all family members, including caregivers, to embrace the 5 Simple Rules.

Parents often ask...

What Rule or Rules should I focus on first?

There is no right answer to this question. It is recommended that you start making the changes that you and your family are ready, willing, and able to make. For help getting started, refer to chapter 2.

Being a role model, or modeling, is intimately connected with just about all of a child's behaviors, including all of the behaviors that are related to weight. For example, toddlers who are picky eaters tend to take after other family members who also are picky eaters. Modeling also has a big effect on activity. In one study of four- to seven-year-olds, those kids with active mothers were twice as likely to be active as those whose mothers were not. When fathers were active, the kids were three and a half times more likely to be active. When both parents were active, the children were almost six times more likely to be active. The researchers believed that modeling was a major factor behind this connection. Because kids learn by what they see, the importance of being a role model cannot be underestimated.

Providing

As providers, we are responsible for providing food, clothing, and shelter for our families. Kids are dependent on us to provide for their needs, including those that affect their weight.

When our children are left with caregivers, the provider role is assumed by them. It helps to know what children are provided with during the time they are with caregivers, as it may not be in line with the 5 Simple Rules. In a survey of caregivers who took care of kids under the age of five, it was discovered that only 46% of nursery schools and 23% of sitters provided a fruit or vegetable with meals. Only 14% of nursery schools and 21% of sitters provided a dairy food, like low-fat milk, with meals every day. While almost all the caregivers saw themselves as having a responsibility in providing wise food choices, they felt that the food guidance that they were provided was too vague. In addition, the caregivers described tension with parents. The researchers concluded that caregivers would benefit from clear directions and expectations about what foods should be served to the children they care for.

Parents often ask . . .

How can I tell my child's caregiver what I want?

As a general rule, the direct approach is best. If you want your child to drink low-fat milk with his meals, say so. Likewise, if after-school television watching is not what you want, you need to give specific instructions. If you want your child to have yogurt or fruit as a snack, you may need to say so and provide them. Children should not and cannot be expected to follow the rules on their own. At the same time, it cannot be assumed that your caregiver will know what you want.

Besides food, children rely on their families for activity. In a study done in the United Kingdom, it was found that many parents are anxious about making decisions about how much freedom their children should have when it comes to being active. This anxiety can be reduced by learning more about the many ways that kids can be active and by creating realistic goals and action plans.

Enforcing

Enforcing the family's rules and regulations is part of being a parent, both an art and a science. Adults, especially those who live in the family home, are the ones who decide the rules that kids must live by. We also are the ones who communicate the expectations in our words and actions (by being a role model). In setting expectations, consider that a child's ability to do what is expected depends on the child's age and thinking skills.

Different homes have different rules, and the number and type of rules affect how a child will react. Children are more likely to follow rules if they anticipate a negative consequence, like a punishment, than if they don't. Conversely, in homes where there are few rules and low expectations, children are less likely to comply.

Adults may set the rules, but that does not mean that the kids always go along. Research suggests that how difficult a specific child is about following house rules stays relatively steady over time, with a peak in early adolescence and a decrease in the late teen years. Studies also show that children who resist rules are more likely to be aggressive and blame their problems on other people. This means that those children who resist house rules, such as curfews and picking up after themselves, are also more likely to resist the 5 Simple Rules. And if these are the same kids who have weight issues, they are likely to blame their excess weight on others. While resistant kids can be a challenge to any parent, the effort put into working issues through is worthwhile.

Consistency matters, with studies showing that inconsistent enforcement of the rules is more likely to cause problems with non-compliance. Likewise, disagreement among the enforcers in the house about how and when to punish a child has been linked with kids not following the rules.

Protecting

As parents, we protect our children. In today's world, the role of protecting our kids has shifted from physical issues like paddling in schools to emotional issues like bullying and feelings of isolation. Emotional problems are the major cause of disability in today's kids. The role of protecting our kids is shared by many, including families, schools, and the government. In a study that looked at this issue in the United Kingdom, it was found that benefits from steps taken to promote the health of our children today may last into adulthood. The study found that providing support to kids at home, having a safe environment to promote activities like walking or biking to school, working for safe neighborhoods, and limiting advertising for treats targeted to kids are effective steps.

Advocating

The *American Heritage Dictionary* defines an advocate as someone who argues for a cause. The argument can take the form of defending the cause or supporting a change. Because children are not in a position to be their own advocates, this is a role that we as parents take on.

As advocates, we can help create a healthy-weight environment for our children outside the home. Changes are often most effective when advocates from different walks of life join together to work for a cause. For example, in a project in Chicago, Illinois, a group that includes researchers, public health officials, and medical professionals joined together to work toward programs geared at preventing childhood over-weight. Dr. Lane France, one of the experts profiled in the introduction to part one, is doing something similar in Tampa, Florida.

Evidence shows that advocacy efforts make a difference. Examples include groups of advocates encouraging schools to add physical education back into their curriculums and a community project that involved nearly a hundred people working to lower fat intake and increase activity among Native American children.

Parents Need to Be Parents

Children thrive on structure. They look to us to set the rules, create the limits, and enforce the rules of the house, everything from curfews to brushing teeth. In creating a healthy-weight home, structure comes from the parenting roles that are used to make the 5 Simple Rules part of the family's life—in other words, incorporating the rules into every part of parenting. Examples include providing a limited supply of treats or deciding that a worthy goal is to have the family spend more time outdoors. Over the course of days, weeks, and years, the rules need to evolve as the children grow older.

As parents, we have the power to change our family's attitudes about health and weight. We are in the best position to shift the family's concern from losing weight to focusing on living a healthy lifestyle. But the responsibility to comply is shared by everyone, including siblings and caregivers. Managing weight is not something that anyone, adults or children, can do alone.

Style Also Counts

Research shows that kids do best when their parents adapt their parenting styles to fit a child's nature, personality, and needs. Children need unconditional love and quality time. An authoritative parenting style balancing warmth and affection with consistent expectations and limits increases the chances of having happy, cooperative, and confident kids. By contrast, studies indicate that parents who are rigid, authoritarian, or permissive are likely to have less success.

Experts recommend that in taking on the various roles of a parent, it is better to guide than to dictate. Guiding food choices helps children learn to make their own decisions rather than simply learn that some foods are okay to eat and others are not. You can spark a child's interest in exercise with encouragement and guidance, by exploring different activity options, supporting participation in the activity, and showing confidence in a child's ability to do the activity.

Functioning as a Family

A child's ability to think and to handle the relationships that are part of life are affected by how well his or her family functions. Research shows that family closeness or togetherness makes a big difference. Members of families that function well feel connected to each other. In these homes, the kids feel close to their parents and to each other. Families are dynamic—parents influence the kids, the parents affect each other, and the children make their parents change and adjust as they grow older. Several studies find that family solidarity is a powerful motivator for changing eating and activity patterns.

Parents often ask . . .

Do I have to be perfect?

Absolutely not! No one is perfect, and having a healthy-weight home is about progress, not perfection. Because there are thousands of food and activity behaviors to choose from, you are able to pick those that are important to you and that you know your family can do.

No one type of family structure is more effective than others. A healthy family can have one or two parents, one child or several children. Children will do well in most family structures as long as the way the family functions is positive and strong.

PART TWO

Family Power

While there are many factors that make the topic of excess weight in children complex, the basics of combating the problem are clear: Understanding and implementing the five parenting roles are the key to creating a healthy-weight home that lives by the 5 Simple Rules. Five roles, five rules.

Why it is important that the entire family live by the Rules and the specific steps that can be taken to make it work are what we discuss in part two.

The Family Power Pilot Project

Weight Watchers is committed to helping people achieve a healthy weight, from the adults of today to the children of future generations.

For the past two years, Weight Watchers International has been piloting a family-based program geared to helping parents create a healthy-weight home. Over the course of eight weekly sessions, the 5 Simple Rules and the roles of role model, provider, enforcer, protector, and advocate have been explored, discussed, and tried. We have had many discussions about the readiness to make changes as well as what changes to try now and what changes to leave for a future date.

The sessions are facilitated by coaches who have received special training in childhood weight issues. The pilot sessions are attended only by the parents, who act as representatives for their family—they come, learn, and discuss and then take the information and ideas home to test out. About a hundred families have participated in the pilot so far and the results have been encouraging.

The next eight chapters take an in-depth look at how each of the five parental roles can be used to make the 5 Simple Rules come alive. Besides presenting the latest scientific findings about effective strategies, each chapter offers insights and experiences from families who have participated in the Weight Watchers pilot. Some of the families have asked to remain anonymous, so their stories are told through the coaches. However, many families wanted to share their experiences directly with you. Their family portraits can be found at the end of each chapter.

Clara Ruggles, Tina Harvey, Kelley Brickfield, and Sue Montegny are coaches for the Family Power pilot. They went through a rigorous selection process to become coaches. Each has had extensive experience in helping adults achieve a healthy weight because they are Weight Watchers Leaders. (Weight Watchers Leaders are people who have achieved and are maintaining a healthy weight themselves by following the Weight Watchers program. After rigorous training, leaders facilitate Weight Watchers meetings, helping others to achieve their weight-loss goals.)

Just being a Weight Watchers Leader, however, did not earn the coaches a spot on the Family Power team. They applied for the special

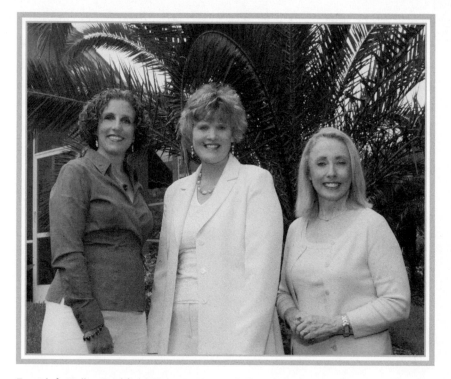

From left, Kelley Brickfield, Tina Harvey, and Clara Ruggles (Sue Montegny was not able to be at the photo shoot)

training and were interviewed before selection. Through the interview process, they demonstrated their commitment to helping families make a healthy-weight home and told of their own journey to make this happen for their families. All four of the coaches have kids of their own and have faced the ups and downs of following the 5 Simple Rules. One is even a grandmother!

Besides bringing to the project their commitment and experience, each coach received extensive training from Weight Watchers International on the science of childhood obesity and the Family Power pilot program. The coaches have put that knowledge into practice, coaching dozens of families—just like yours—in the 5 Simple Rules and how to be an effective role model, provider, enforcer, protector, and advocate. In their sessions, they have learned a great deal—what works and what doesn't work, how to overcome resistance, and when to push forward and when to let go.

One of the key lessons that the coaches have learned is that a healthy-weight home is about progress, not perfection. Every family they have coached has been able to make some changes. While some have made more than others, everyone has spoken of a change that has made a difference in the health and happiness of their family.

Chapter 6

The Kids Are Watching

One of the most important roles—if not the most important—we as parents play is to be a role model. Being a role model is the doing part of being a parent. Like it or not, kids watch what we do and learn from it. Children learn positive behaviors, like having good table manners and saying please and thank you, and they can learn negative behaviors, like cursing. We don't have a choice about being a role model. We do have a lot of choice, however, about the kind of role model we want to be. Because being a role model is so important, the next two chapters will explore the role in detail. This chapter deals with being a food role model, including the story of three generations of the Ruggles family. The ins and outs of being an activity role model are discussed in chapter 7.

What Is a Food Role Model?

Parents are a child's first and most powerful role models when it comes to food, including what, when, and how much to eat. Besides modeling specific food choices, parents also model their attitudes, values, and beliefs about food and eating. For example, if you believe that eating a wholesome breakfast is important and eat one every day, most likely your kids will too.

> ### Good Food Role Models
> - Eat wholesome, nutritious foods
> - Enjoy treats in moderation
> - Make family meals a time for togetherness
> - Show that healthy eating is part of feeling good about and taking care of yourself

Being a good role model for food and eating is following the 5 Simple Rules consistently and with a positive attitude. In creating a healthy-weight home, we take on the responsibility for family eating. Researchers describe this as parents working side by side with each other and with their children, without blame or scolding, to practice healthy eating. Role modeling gives the chance to show by example that working toward a healthy weight is a valuable part of daily life. Following the 5 Simple Rules by making the recommended food and activity choices shows kids that we parents have a positive opinion of ourselves, and this helps kids have strong feelings of self-worth.

Being a food role model covers a lot of ground and includes many small behaviors. It means being on center stage when it comes to eating, including what foods are eaten, how foods are combined into meals and snacks, and how much food to eat. Each one of these small behaviors, plus many more, adds up to teach children most of what they know about food and eating.

Many strategies can be used to create and maintain Rules #1 and #2. As with all of the roles, the strategies vary according to the child's age, with different recommendations for infants, toddlers and young children, and older children.

Infants

Infants do not talk, but they keep a close eye on what is going on around them. In particular, they watch what their parents, their caregivers, and other kids are doing. Although a baby's food is limited to either breast milk or formula for about the first six months of life, babies are already learning eating habits before taking their first bite of food.

What works for infants is making them a part of family meals as soon as they are settled into a feeding routine. Working into a feeding schedule with a newborn can be tough for the first month or so, but most infants get into a routine fairly quickly. It helps to try to get the baby on a feeding schedule that does not overlap with family meals.

Infants get their first lessons in how to eat by watching the people around them. This usually means parents and other family members. Babies become curious about the foods they see being eaten around them. In fact, one way to tell that a baby is ready to start solids is a growing interest in family foods. Some infants grab at the foods others are eating. Most infants are ready to start solids around their six-month birthday.

Coach's Corner — Learning how to eat

Situation: A mother had questions for me about her ten-month-old son who loved his bottle but had no interest in eating solid foods.

Strategies: In discussing the situation with her, I discovered that her son had not had a lot of opportunities to watch other people eating. The family routine was to feed the baby before eating and then have him take a nap or play in another room while the family sat down for meals. As a result, he did not sit at the table during family mealtimes. We did not know if this was playing into her son's lack of interest in food, but we decided to try an experiment. For the next week, the routine was changed. The baby joined the family for meals, getting his bottle while everyone else ate. As the days went by, he watched everyone else eating and enjoying their food. Then he started to take less interest in his bottle and more interest in food. Within weeks, the baby had taken his place at the family table and was eating the same foods as his brother and sisters.

Having enjoyable family meals means more than just having good table manners. It includes a pleasant mealtime atmosphere with a routine that includes things like sitting at a table, using utensils to eat, having friendly conversation, and focusing on each other without distractions like a television.

Meals that include a variety of foods teach kids of all ages about the concept of a balanced diet and show the importance of eating foods from all the food groups. Because babies are interested in family foods from a very young age, they learn what a meal looks like—different colors and shapes of food—even though they may be too young to know what the foods are and are not able to taste them.

Once babies move away from baby foods, they can eat the same foods as the rest of the family. Even at this young age, kids catch on quickly if they think they are being manipulated to get them to eat something. Trilling "This broccoli is *sooooo* good!" and then grimacing when the broccoli comes to the table sends a clear message that something is not right and this food is not to be trusted. Making a big deal about a food with either words or body language affects a child's beliefs and preferences for that food, both positively and negatively. It does not take long for a child to figure out that the *"Yum!"* that comes with ice cream and the frown that comes with spinach means that ice cream is something you want and spinach is not. For this reason, experts recommend keeping neutral and equal reactions to all foods.

What doesn't work is forcing babies to eat. Research indicates that infants who are encouraged or coaxed to finish a bottle or meal or to eat if they are not hungry are more likely to gain excess weight over time. Not only does this habit encourage babies to take in more calories than their bodies need, it can disrupt their learning the natural signals of fullness and hunger by encouraging them to overeat when they are young. In turn, this may affect the infant's ability to eat the right amounts of food as he or she grows and develops.

As soon as the infant starts eating solid food, attention to Rule #1—focus on wholesome, nutritious foods—should kick in. For example, babies should be fed prepared baby foods that have been made without added fat or sugar. Making the food at home by pureeing wholesome foods and freezing them in ice cube trays to be used as needed is also an option. Buying prepared baby foods with added sugar or fat may promote a preference for high-calorie, low-nutrient foods later on.

It is also never too early to provide a pleasant eating atmosphere. Even during the very early months when some of the baby's meals are not taken with the family, it helps for whoever is doing the feeding to concentrate on the meal without being distracted by television or loud music. It is not only the person who is doing the feeding who can be distracted. The baby can be too, and these distractions can encourage overeating because attention is taken away from food, and the signs that signal fullness can be missed. Making this a habit helps to set up the infant's natural progression to family meals.

Toddlers and Young Children

Toddlers and young children are highly impressionable. As parents, we are their world, and they want to be just like us in every way.

What works for toddlers and young children is family meals that offer the chance to practice social skills and develop bonds with other family members. Meals without television and other distractions encourage conversation among family members. They also help young kids to focus on what they are eating, to eat more slowly, and to pay attention to their body's hunger and fullness signals. Research shows that children who eat meals with their family, especially dinners, also are more likely to have diets with more nutrients and fewer calories.

Young children are naturally *neophobic*, meaning that they avoid new things. One of the most obvious areas of neophobia is food. A young child typically has an emphatic *No!* to new foods. It is not uncommon for kids to be labeled as picky eaters, and this can set up a situation where the child's food preferences are catered to in order to avoid conflict.

It helps to know that virtually all children, left to their own devices, will become picky eaters. This need not be the case, however, because the way new foods are introduced can help lessen food neophobia. Research finds that it may take between ten and fourteen exposures to a new food for a child to feel brave enough to eat it. That means that a useful strategy is to keep serving and eating the same food day after day, but without making a big deal about it. Keep the faith that, in time and without prodding, the child will try it. It helps if others are eating the food at the same time and with a no-big-deal attitude. Seeing others eating a new food takes away some of the fear factor for a young child.

Even after repeated exposure to a food over a few days, a young child simply will not like certain foods. This does not mean, however, that it is not a good idea to try the same food again when the child is a few months older. In one study that looked at how kids increased the variety of foods that they ate over time, it was found that those who learned to eat a variety of vegetables and dairy foods as young children were more likely to eat a wide variety of foods in later years. The most important factor, however, was a child's exposure to foods before the age of four.

Coach's Corner
Overcoming a past of picky eating

Situation: I was talking to a couple who described themselves as being picky eaters when they were kids. They wanted to know what steps they might try to keep their young daughter, who was just entering the "terrible twos," from being the same way.

Strategies: We explored different ways that they could be food role models and help their daughter avoid the food fears that often lead to picky eating. One strategy we discussed was to mix things up at the barbecue. Dad did a lot of grilling, and the family had settled into a routine of having only a few grilled items like chicken and trout. He decided to expand his cooking to include a variety of fishes as well as poultry and meat. He also began to grill vegetables like peppers, asparagus, summer squash, and eggplant. Because his daughter was used to eating things right off her Dad's grill, she was more willing to try these new foods. Mom also wanted to help her daughter eat yogurt. To help this along, she would have an afternoon snack of yogurt and share bites with her daughter. While not every grilled food or flavor of yogurt was accepted by their daughter, the couple was convinced that these strategies were helping her to try new foods and not become a picky eater.

Research finds that many parents don't realize that young children who are old enough to handle a spoon are old enough to feed themselves. And while letting young children feed themselves is often a hassle because it takes so long and makes a mess, it is an important strategy to use. Not only does it encourage physical skills and coordination, but letting children feed themselves small portions—as little as a tablespoon or two of each food per year of age—helps them to eat the calories their body needs without overeating. This is especially true for treats, like ice cream or cookies. Giving small portions and letting them feed themselves gives young children the pleasure of eating treats without too many calories.

Another good strategy for many families with young children and toddlers is to offer an ever-expanding choice of wholesome foods. As described in the 5 Simple Rules, focusing on wholesome, nutritious meals and snacks is an important part of having a healthy-weight home. When it comes to snacks, it is not uncommon to get in a rut and have the same foods all the time. Providing different food options for snacks is an easy way to expose young children to new foods, especially since small kids need snacks throughout the day to get the calories they need. Keeping treats separate from snacks is also a recommended strategy. Young children do not know the nutritional value or caloric content of foods—they learn what to eat from us.

(Coach's Corner)   **Making the move to treats**

Situation: A parent asked me for advice on changing the types of foods in the house—focusing more on wholesome foods and reducing the amount of cookies and candy in the kitchen cupboard. A big concern was how the children would react to the change and whether it would lead to food fights.

Strategies: This parent's timing was excellent because the children were young and likely to accept food changes without asking too many questions. I suggested avoiding any mention to the children of the disappearance of the cookies and candies. Also, we discussed not calling attention to new foods like whole-grain cereals and frozen fruit bars. Once the new foods were in the house, family meals and snacks included those foods. As hoped, the children did not really notice the difference. When they asked "Can I have a cookie?" the response "We don't have any right now, so how about an apple with a slice of cheese instead?" was accepted without much trouble at all.

What doesn't work is inconsistency. Despite parents' efforts to focus on wholesome, nutritious foods and include treats in moderation, young children and toddlers soon discover that they like treats and will ask for more. While it is often tempting to give in to the request, it is not a good idea. Research shows that providing treats in an irregular or unpredictable way is likely to reinforce a child's preference for these foods. This is true whether the parents are eating the food or not. On the flip side, rigid restrictions and a pointed avoidance of those foods does not work well either. The best strategy is to include the foods as the child's choice of treats, thereby teaching the child about the place treats can have as part of a healthy diet.

Using favorite foods as a reward or gift, as well as taking them away as a punishment, is a common tactic to make a child behave. When it comes to having a healthy-weight home, this tactic is not helpful.

(Coach's Corner)   **When rigid rules backfire**

Situation: A mother and father came to me with a dilemma. They wanted to improve the eating habits of their children and had decided that foods made with white flour or sugar would not be allowed in the house. This meant that cupcakes, ice cream, candy, and a lot of other foods were forbidden. Also as part of this restriction, the parents had created a rule that it was okay to eat the cheese topping from the pizza but not the crust. At parties and away from home, however, their young children stuffed themselves on pizza with crust, cupcakes, and other foods they were forbidden to eat at home. Clearly, the strategy was not working.

Strategies: I explained to the parents that extreme rules can bring negative consequences and that is exactly what they were seeing in their kids. We discussed the difference between rigid restrictions and more sensible guidelines that include some treats. While this was difficult for them to accept, they decided to experiment by letting go of the no-crust rule on pizza. That week, the parents ordered a pizza for dinner, told the kids it was okay to eat the crust now, and they ate the crust too. Over time, they saw that when their kids were at a pizza party, they were not as likely to overeat the pizza, but instead were satisfied with a slice. This experiment helped the parents to see that they had been too rigid with their food rules.

Research finds that rewarding healthy eating with treats teaches children that certain foods are more desirable than others. It is also a common strategy to offer dessert on the condition that a child eat vegetables, or to make a child eat a certain number of bites to get dessert. This practice sends a clear message to the child: dessert is better than wholesome foods.

While meals that provide wholesome, nutritious foods are a key ingredient in creating a healthy-weight home, forcing anyone to eat a specific food or to eat a designated amount of food is not helpful. Attempting to be a role model for healthy eating by eating foods that you really dislike is unlikely to be successful. Moreover, forcing a child to eat is not good for the parent-child relationship and sets up food as a battleground.

A good strategy to follow is that the parents are responsible for deciding which foods to serve, while each family member has the responsibility for deciding what and how much to eat. Young children who stop eating during a meal or who say that they do not want to eat probably are not hungry and so should not be encouraged to eat. Also, growth slows after infancy, and young kids may eat less food than they did when they were younger.

Research shows that most young children and toddlers eat only one "good" meal per day and that's enough. Young children may also choose to eat only one or two foods at each meal (parents usually eat at least three or four different foods). That's okay too. As a parent, you can show your children that to stop eating when you're full is the right thing to do by sometimes leaving food on your plate.

Older Children

Older children who spend more time away from home are more independent in their food choices. Many purchase snack foods and occasional meals for themselves. Despite their growing independence, older children continue to be influenced by their parents' example when it comes to food and eating.

What works for older children is regular family meals. Eating together as a family sends an important message to older children. Children learn to value family time when they are asked to sit down together and eat with their parents and siblings no matter how busy the family schedule is. And being role models for the 5 Simple Rules shows older children that family meals are part of daily life. A pleasant meal environment also can help older children relax and open up about what is going on in their lives.

As children grow older, it remains the parents' job to decide what foods are provided and when meals will be served. Older children should be encouraged to serve themselves from the foods that are provided and to decide how much to eat. Research shows that children who serve themselves tend to take smaller portions.

Watching their parents as positive role models, older children may begin to appreciate that eating a lot of treats, such as chips, candy, cookies, and soft drinks, can lead to excess weight and that focusing on wholesome, nutritious foods aids in weight management. A strategy that works for some families is to encourage *treat boredom* by buying only one type of cookie or salty snack. That way, the treats are available but not too enticing.

Coach's Corner   Making treats work

Situation: A mother came to me with a dilemma. She had a weight issue herself and said that her weakness was cookies. She wanted to be a good role model for her kids, who had asked for cookies as one of their treat foods, but was concerned about her ability to keep any cookies in the house without overeating them herself.

Strategies: In discussing the situation, we discovered that the children enjoyed fig bars but that they were the one cookie that Mom could take or leave. With this in mind, Mom decided to purchase fig bars to use as a treat. When I checked back with her a few weeks later, Mom reported that the strategy was working for both her and her kids. The kids enjoyed having their cookie treat, and when Mom really wanted a cookie, she found that she could eat a fig bar and enjoy it without fear of eating the whole package.

Family traditions like Sunday lunch after church, Saturday morning family breakfast, and special holiday meals enhance the joy of eating. New traditions can make meals as a family something to look forward to.

Coach's Corner **New traditions**

Situation: In the spring, a father and I were talking about how Easter had become a day of overeating in his home. From candy in the Easter baskets to ham-with-all-the-fixings dinner and dessert, he was looking for ways to make this year different. Since his two children were preteens, he wondered whether he should sit down with them to discuss other options that might help promote a healthy-weight home.

Strategies: With my encouragement, Dad called a family meeting and asked his kids for ideas for new Easter traditions that would not take the celebration away from the holiday. He, his wife, and their two children decided to start a tradition of making the day an outdoor outing to enjoy the spring weather. The whole family prepared the traditional Easter ham and fixings on Saturday evening and refrigerated everything. On Easter morning, Mom and Dad packed a picnic lunch and took the kids to a local theme park for the day. The day was proclaimed a success because they ate less than they would have at home and got a lot of exercise walking around the park. When asked, the kids were very positive about the outing, even suggesting that next year's destination be the zoo.

Being a food role model is not limited to what goes on at home. Older children in particular watch how their parents make food choices when the family is eating out. Research shows that super-sized meals and large portions encourage kids to eat more. In one study, children who were served a double-sized portion took larger bites and ate more calories. When parents order these meals, it sends the message to their children that these amounts of food are appropriate.

Once older children can read and understand nutrition information on menus and online, they may be interested in discussing what they have learned. While it is not possible to decide what teens will eat when they are away from home, helping them to be informed and sharing nutrition information helps.

> **Coach's Corner** **Fast food**
>
> **Situation:** One of the mothers I worked with was proud that her teenage son plays after-school sports. She admitted that she often takes the family for a fast-food meal on the way home from his practices since they end so late. Because her son is so active physically, she did not want to restrict what he chooses, even though she may not agree with his choices.
>
> **Strategies:** We decided that it would not be helpful for Mom to comment on her son's food choices, even if he picks the biggest burger on the menu. However, I mentioned that she should set an example by ordering wholesome foods for herself. With this in mind, Mom became very aware of her own food choices when they ate fast food, consistently ordering a grilled chicken sandwich, a salad with low-fat dressing, a baked potato, and the like. Over time and much to her surprise, she found that her son began to order some of these items as well. He didn't order them all the time, but he often did because he found that he liked them and it gave him an alternative to his usual burger and fries.

What we as parents do ourselves sets the stage for what our children do, often without our even realizing the impact. One example is snacking in front of the television. Research shows that parents who are in the habit of snacking in front of the television raise children who are likely to do the same. It has also been found that older children who nibble while watching television are likely to eat without being fully aware of what and how much they have eaten. Children who eat and watch television often eat more calories than they would if the television were off. Eating in front of the television can be a particularly troubling habit with older children in the after-school hours. Limiting screen time and, if possible, having a house rule of not eating in front of the television is a good strategy for the entire family.

Coach's Corner   Learning portion sizes

Situation: One mother and father reported to me that the family pediatrician said that all three of their sons needed to make better food choices because they were gaining too much weight. Their biggest problem was eating large portions, especially of salty snacks, cookies, and frozen meals. The boys had no idea of what is considered an appropriate portion size and were unaware that the amounts of foods they were eating were a major factor in their weight gain.

Strategies: Because the two older boys were old enough to understand the basic concepts of label reading, I suggested that Dad show them how he reads the Nutrition Facts panel to understand serving sizes and to be more aware of the amounts of food that he eats. With Dad as a role model, his sons became very conscious of what they were eating. They started reading every nutrition label, telling their Dad what they had found out and what they thought about it. This started an ongoing discussion about portion sizes and how, by reading labels, you can get more food for the calories by choosing one food over another. Dad believed these discussions were helping his boys to make more informed food choices.

When children see parents use food to calm and comfort themselves, they learn that food can be a powerful coping mechanism. They also learn to eat outside of regularly scheduled meals and snacks when they feel stressed. However, seeing parents who have learned to handle stress and emotional ups and downs through other means, including physical activity, private time, and nonfood rewards, helps children learn nonfood coping skills, an important predictor of lasting weight management.

The Ruggles Family Story

by Clara Ruggles

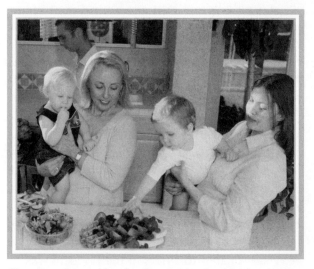

Clara Ruggles and her family enjoying healthy food

I am living proof that being a role model works. Because I have worked so hard to be a positive role model for my kids, they do not have the same weight issues I had as a child. It is especially rewarding that my grandkids do not have weight issues either.

How could this be when I have generations of heavy relatives? I think the answer is that I broke the family cycle of Midwest country cooking traditions. My parents and grandparents served mostly fried foods topped with gravy. We ate lots of potatoes and gravy at every meal, even breakfast. It is no surprise that everyone in my family was overweight. My kids entered this world with the odds stacked against them. Children who have at least one obese parent are more likely to have weight problems as well.

After my second child was born, I decided to challenge my own fate and try to lose weight. I joined Weight Watchers just for me without realizing what a difference it could make in the weight of my children. I was in charge of buying and preparing food for the family, so I bought what I needed to eat, and my husband and two young children ate what I ate. I didn't prepare special foods for them. You could say that I was an accidental role model because I wasn't trying to be one; it just happened.

It took a long time for my kids to realize that the foods they ate at home were different from the foods that other families were eating. It was hard to know what to say when my kids came home from their friends' houses. After one sleepover, my son told me that his friend's mom served doughnuts for breakfast. I didn't want to get into a big discussion or fight about doughnuts so I just said, "Really? Doughnuts? That's different."

My children benefited because I learned to prepare foods differently from the way foods were prepared when I was a child. No frying—I broiled or baked foods—and no gravy and no piles of potatoes. I dished out modest portions for my kids when they were younger. Once they were older, I put food out on the counter and we all served ourselves. They learned how much to take by watching me. Keeping food on the counter instead of on the table helped all of us avoid taking seconds or picking at the leftovers.

When it came to treats in the house, I was the role model. There were very few treats for me and very few for the kids. My kids never became big snack food eaters, because snacks were not in the house. They knew that they could eat fruit anytime they were hungry.

Both of my children are adults now and I am a proud mother and grandmother. My daughter and son never had weight issues. They focus on wholesome, nutritious foods and both belong to health clubs so that they get regular physical activity. My grandchildren are very healthy eaters who love vegetables and fruits.

I broke the chain of excess weight in my family. By being a role model for a healthy lifestyle, I helped my children and my grandchildren live healthier lives and avoid the need to deal with excess weight.

Chapter 7

Active Parents, Active Kids

Just as we are role models for food, we are role models for activity. There are differences, though. When it comes to food, everybody eats, and it becomes a matter of what children see when it comes to food and eating behaviors. For activity, role modeling is more a matter of *if there is activity* as opposed to what is being done. This chapter looks at how our kids are affected by whether and how we move and includes a profile of the Von Dolteren family, who showcase the idea of being activity role models.

What Is an Activity Role Model?

According to Healthy People 2010, a government-recommended game plan to improve the health of Americans, close to half of American adults do not get any leisure-time physical activity. This trend to be sedentary is having major health consequences, including higher rates of overweight and obesity. Inactivity is so harmful to health that one of the goals for the Healthy People 2010 project is to cut in half the number of adults who are not physically active.

Children need positive role models for activity both inside and outside the home. As parents, we are the primary role models. Children learn by watching how we spend our free time—from watching television to taking a walk to visiting the gym a few times a week.

> ### Good Activity Role Models
>
> - Are active
> - Strive to get some structured exercise
> - Reduce screen time
> - Plan family outings that include activity
> - Get at least sixty minutes of activity each day

Being an activity role model means being active yourself by looking for ways to make moving a part of your day, several times each day. For most of us, this means being more aware of the opportunities to be active and then taking the time to do so. Kids will get active when they are included as part of the activity routines of others. Small steps that help you get daily activity include always taking the stairs instead of an escalator or elevator at stores, office buildings, and the like; consistently pulling into parking spaces that are a distance from a store's entrance and then walking to the store; unfailingly walking the dog a few times a day; and using a push mower to cut the grass.

Truly active adults also make time for some kind of planned exercise: a daily brisk walk, a class at the health club or gym, time on the treadmill, or participation in an organized team for golf, volleyball, softball, or basketball.

Because limiting screen time is one of the Rules for a healthy-weight home, this is a particularly important area for role models. Strong messages are sent to kids about their own screen time when they see the adults in the home reducing their own time watching television and surfing the Internet. In today's world, it is common for all of us, not just kids, to spend hours each day in screen time at home.

Coach's Corner — Parents need to walk the talk

Situation: A mother and father proudly told me that they wanted to cut down their children's screen time so they took the televisions out of the preteen's bedrooms. They kept the television in the master bedroom, however, because they did not see it as a problem and, when their kids complained that this was unfair, said that this was not a change that they were willing to do themselves.

Strategies: I explained that they were sending their kids mixed messages because they were saying one thing (having a television in your bedroom is not okay) and doing another (having a television in my bedroom is okay). If they supported the idea that the 5 Simple Rules apply to everyone, they needed to make a choice. They chose to allow televisions in all the bedrooms for now and focus working on other changes in the home that they could and would do as well.

Powerful role models take the time freed by reducing screen time and use it for some type of physical activity. According to the 2005 Dietary Guidelines for Americans, to get the health benefits of activity like lower blood pressure and reduced stress levels, adults need thirty daily minutes of moderate to vigorous activity. The guidelines go on to say, however, that thirty minutes is not enough to prevent weight gain or maintain a weight loss. If a healthy-weight home is a goal, more activity is needed. The guidelines recommend sixty minutes of activity a day both for adults who want to avoid gaining weight and for all children regardless of weight. For adults who have lost weight and want to keep it off, studies show that sixty to ninety minutes per day of activity are needed.

Many people are put off by these recommendations because they seem unattainable. With our busy lives, finding an hour a day for our children and ourselves to be active can seem impossible. A closer look at the guidelines, however, brings the recommendations into a more realistic view. The recommendations are based on accumulated activity and include activities that can be part of daily life. This means that walking the dog with your child, dashing as a family from the far end of the parking lot to the store, and taking the stairs to get to the third-floor pediatrician's office translate into minutes of activity. Making the most of opportunities to move throughout the day helps make the recommendations possible. Being an activity role model to your kids is one of the best legacies that you can give them.

The Benefits of Physical Activity

Becoming active is one of the healthiest things that any family can do— there are more benefits linked to being active than you can get from making just about any other change in the way you live. There is no doubt that a key benefit of activity is weight management. Research shows that a lack of physical activity is one of the major factors behind childhood overweight, and activity helps prevent a child from having weight issues. Regular activity also builds muscles, and because muscles burn calories 24/7, they boost metabolism. Finally, activity helps reduce how much fat is carried on a child's body.

Physical activity improves overall health and well-being. It helps to build strong bones in children and may lessen their chances of having weak bones as adults. Adults who are physically active have a lower chance of developing heart disease, diabetes, and certain cancers. Physical activity improves our mood and helps us cope with stress.

As with most lifestyle changes, activity should be increased in small and gradual steps. Taking small steps, first to be more active and then to exercise more, is more likely to lead to lasting changes for adults and kids alike. This approach is especially good for children because it helps them to develop patterns that will stay with them into adulthood.

Most kids do not get the recommended amount of daily activity, and the world we live in is making the problem worse. As discussed in part one, many schools have cut down on physical education classes and the time allowed for recess, many neighborhoods are not designed for kids to be playing outside, and the amount of time a typical child spends in front of screens is on the rise.

Active adults inspire kids to make being active a part of their day. They show that activity is important and worth the time and effort. In addition, role models prove that it is possible. Research shows that children are more likely to take part in and enjoy activity when their parents do too. Kids feel particularly good about activity when they get encouragement. Combined with a focus on wholesome, nutritious foods, regular activity shifts the calorie balance in a way that helps stop weight gain and supports growing into a child's weight.

An added benefit to being active for all family members is the likelihood that mindless snacking will be reduced. Both children and adults often eat without thinking when they are watching television, working on the computer, or playing video games. Snacking is also a common

---

Coach's Corner   The computer-snack cycle

Situation: One of the mothers I work with was concerned because her teenage son spent hours at the computer and playing video games. To add to her concern, her son snacked nonstop on whatever was in the house while he sat at the computer or in front of the video console.

Strategies: As Mom and I talked about her son, she discovered that she, too, was in the habit of having a lot of screen time. She agreed to make a concerted effort to both cut back on her own screen time and spend time outside every day. I suggested that she encourage her son to join her. At first, he preferred to stay inside. With encouragement, however, he began to come outside for a few minutes as a way to take a break. As the days went on, the outside visits grew longer. Being outside gave him an opportunity to meet other kids in the neighborhood who asked him to join them in their outside activities. He agreed. Having a choice, he picked being outside with friends over playing on the computer. And because he was outside playing, his snacking also decreased.

response to boredom. When the family is active, children are less likely to be bored, to snack, and to turn to screens.

Infants

Infants are not active in the true sense of the word. Particularly for the first six months, babies are not able to move very far. This does not mean, however, that they are not aware of the activity going on around them. Physical skills begin to develop in infancy and are affected by the way infants are held, the types of toys they are provided, and their sur-roundings—colorful mobiles to look at, music to listen and dance to, and lots of play time with everyone in the family. During this vital time of development, babies learn how to move and be active by exploring their world and by playing.

What works during infancy is simple types of play that get the baby moving. During the first couple of months, this can include wiggling the legs and arms or offering a finger or toy for the infant to grab. "Mommy and me" classes offer exercise for mothers—some classes include exer-cises that can be done with a stroller so the babies see their mothers being active. A walk in the park or through the neighborhood with a baby in a stroller or baby carrier gives the infant a chance to observe the world. The American Academy of Pediatrics and others recommend that infants have at least one hour daily of active playtime.

What doesn't work is having an infant spend a lot of time being inactive. It is helpful to be aware of how much time a baby spends in an infant seat, swing, crib, or playpen. This includes when the baby is in the hands of a caregiver. Limiting the amount of time spent in a con-fined space encourages babies to move around and be active, and this also helps them to develop.

Toddlers and Young Children

Once children start to walk, the size of their world greatly expands. It is during these early years that toddlers and young children learn all the basic physical skills that they need for activity, including walking, running, hopping, skipping, throwing, catching, kicking, and balancing. Having role models as these skills are being learned helps a lot. Children who are encouraged to be active and who play often with family and friends become more coordinated. It is more fun for kids to take part in activities when they have good physical skills.

What works for toddlers and young children is seeing those around them being active, including older siblings. With both eating and activity, young children learn by watching others. Having active role models increases children's *self-efficacy*—their confidence in being able to perform a skill—and tells the child that activity is important.

Every family member is a role model for a young child, so family-centered activities are a boost. Family activities also improve everybody's health and show that exercise is important not just if you are overweight. Children learn that being active is fun, no matter what your age or size.

Coach's Corner — Activity for all

Situation: A family with five school-age children had very busy lives. Without their really being aware of it, their lifestyle had developed into one where they never did family-based activities. The children pursued their own activities on an irregular basis and the parents were sedentary.

Strategies: Mom realized that their lifestyle was not helping their weight and they were not developing the family closeness that was important to her. We explored options that the whole family could enjoy, and Mom came up with the idea of a family field day at a local park. She planned different activities so that each family member could participate in something. The kids ended up really enjoying the day of games and laughter and asked if the family could do it again soon.

Activity role models teach young children the games that will help them to play with other kids. For example, young children can play the simple outdoor games that all kids love, including hide-and-seek, tag, and kick the can. Children at this age love to show off, and because they enjoy the games, they are likely to play longer when others join in.

As with activity at any age, a stepwise increase in the amount of time spent in active play is recommended. It is tough for young children to go suddenly from no activity to a lot of activity. Not only do small steps help build feelings of self-confidence and pleasure for a child, they are the best way to create activity patterns that will last. At this age, small steps add up to big change.

Coach's Corner — Small steps

Situation: A father was telling me about his young child, who was not very active. She did not have a lot of energy to play because of her excess weight, and this was made worse because she also had poor stamina from being so inactive.

Strategies: We discussed the benefits of taking a gradual approach rather than trying to do a lot at one time. Dad chose to try one new activity each week and to do the activity together with his daughter. One week they played outside together for an afternoon; the next week they rode bikes together. Over the next few months, the child's endurance grew. She became more energetic, and while she began to be more active on her own, she continued to look forward to her weekly afternoon with Dad.

When there are young children in the house, it is especially important to limit screen time for the entire family. Television viewing is the one behavior most strongly linked to weight gain in childhood. It is difficult, if not impossible, to keep a young child away from the television if other family members are watching. Young children are less apt to miss television if they are provided with alternatives that include the whole family.

Just spending more time outdoors automatically increases physical activity. Young children are more motivated to go outside if we join them. Activities for families of young children include hiking, playing on riding toys, biking on tricycles or bicycles, and roller skating. Young children often enjoy helping with outdoor chores like washing the car, walking the dog, going to the mailbox, planting seeds in a garden, sweeping the porch, and raking leaves. Trips to a nature center or an animal farm involve plenty of walking. The key word for young children is *fun*.

Coach's Corner   **Parent as playmate**

Situation: One of the mothers in my class realized how important it is for her to be an activity role model, but she believed that this meant she had to sign up for an exercise class, which she did not want to do. While she was making a lot of headway changing her family's food choices, she was struggling to find ways to work on activity.

Strategies: We talked about how activity could include a lot of different things: playing outside with the kids, taking family walks, waterskiing, and even tossing water balloons and playing tag on the front lawn. Mom knew that she could do these things and have fun too. The kids love having their Mom spend time outside with them. They get a special kick when Mom joins them on the trampoline.

As stand-ins, caregivers also need to understand the importance of activity in a child's day and their job as a role model. Some experts suggest considering whether or not a potential caregiver will support activity and have the space and equipment for it when making decisions about childcare.

What doesn't work is not being active yourself but only talking the talk. Examples include watching television but telling kids not to, sitting in the house but sending the children outside, and avoiding exercise but signing the children up for classes and team sports. Children need role models if the goal is to make being active a habit that will last. An inactive role model sends the message that it is important to be active as a child but not as an adult.

Part of being an activity role model is the words used when playing with the kids. Criticism can discourage a child's desire to be involved. By contrast, praise and positive statements help to motivate a child to continue and further develop skills. During this stage of a child's development, support and encouragement build self-esteem and give the child confidence to keep trying to get better.

Older Children

As children grow older, their activity role models continue to be a major influence on the level of activity they get. Older children are sharp observers and notice whether or not we play with the family and take part in our own adult activities. By participating in physical activity (e.g., biking, hiking, playing basketball or baseball, or going to an exercise class) with or without the kids, we demonstrate the importance of being active, and older children see that we think exercise is fun.

What works for older children is seeing their parents change their behavior and become more active to set a good example. Research finds that the children of active parents tend to be more active; role modeling is linked to higher levels of activity in both children and teens and in both boys and girls. In contrast, the same studies find that children whose parents are sedentary are more likely to stay inside rather than being outside.

Coach's Corner   **From indoors to**
outdoors

Situation: A mom and dad admitted to me that they enjoy a few hours of television after their busy days. Their young daughter was the only family member who would rather play outside than watch television, but often she stayed inside to be with her parents.

Strategies: To their credit, Mom and Dad realized that their television watching was not only preventing them from being positive role models, it was discouraging their daughter from being as active as she wanted to be. We discussed how important it was to make a change in their activity habits and cut down on their screen time. It helped when we discussed that the evening activities did not have to be particularly strenuous; the parents just needed to do something instead of television. Mom and Dad decided that they would insist that the entire family go outside a couple of evenings a week to play basketball, ride bicycles, or hit tennis balls against a backboard. By doing it a few times a week, they were still able to watch television on the evenings when their favorite shows were on. This made them happy, and their young daughter was also happy with the change in the family's routine.

Older children tend to be very busy with school, after-school clubs and lessons, and homework. Unless physical education is part of the school day, a day could easily go by without any activity. Activity role models show kids that, despite being busy, it is possible to make the time to be active. Physical activity is easiest to do when it is part of the daily routine. If activity is incorporated into a child's day-to-day lifestyle, it is likely to remain a part of it going forward.

Today's world is filled with time-saving and energy-saving tools that reduce our need to move, including remote controls, cordless phones,

Making the time

Situation: A mother of elementary school–age and preteen boys commented to me that her children were not very active because their school did not offer many opportunities and choices. She wanted help in finding ways to add small amounts of activity to their day.

Strategies: One idea she loved was scheduling time once a week for the family to exercise to a video. The boys helped pick out the ones that they thought they would enjoy, from kickboxing to dancing to the oldies. She and the boys exercise to a video at least once a week and have a lot of fun. The boys in particular like seeing Mom let her hair down as they dance around the living room.

and automatic garage door openers. For many of us, it is possible to put activity back into the mix by bicycling to a friend's home instead of driving, working in the garden, and looking for other family-friendly opportunities that incorporate exercise. Walking together to or from school adds activity and gives us a chance to spend extra time with the kids.

Dad's challenge

Situation: During a conversation about adding activity to the daily routine, a father told me that he wanted to encourage his family to avoid conveniences like elevators and escalators.

Strategies: He did not need much help from me in coming up with great ideas. He created competitions for the family when shopping on weekends and when on vacation to see who could take the most steps the fastest. The family now takes stairs when at a hotel or an amusement park and when shopping at a mall. He told me that he thinks the kids' energy levels have improved, and now they automatically head for the stairs when they are out.

Coach's Corner **A family event**

Situation: A mom and dad asked me about ways that their family could be more involved in community activities.

Strategies: I told them which area newspapers and Web sites have information on activities for families. They found out about a 5K race and children's race that was to be held in a nearby town on an upcoming Saturday morning. They arrived at the race at six in the morning to sign up and enjoy the prerace excitement. All four family members finished the course and plan to do it again next year.

In many families, the hours after dinner are devoted to television, but limiting screen time to two hours or less per day is a key rule for a healthy-weight home. Adding a family activity after dinner—walking the dog, riding bicycles, or shooting hoops—offers an alternative to watching television. It does not have to happen all at once. There can be a gradual change in the amount of television watched in the evening, for example, by taking an after-dinner walk before sitting down to watch. Older children enjoy being active with others—parents, other adults, neighbors, teachers, and friends. Fun is contagious. A family soccer or softball game quickly can grow into a neighborhood tradition.

What doesn't work for older children is a lack of support. For kids, this means not having activity role models, spending time with adults who do not take an interest in their activities, or being criticized for their efforts. These kids are at risk of being turned off to activity for good. While they may not say it, older children need support.

Older children often prefer a looser activity schedule. They may not enjoy strictly defined activities with a tight schedule. Playing with friends or family—a casual basketball game, tossing a ball, riding bikes around the neighborhood, or going for a swim—can be more enjoyable than structured team sports. Even without being influenced by today's fast-paced movies, television shows, computer games, and music, older children prefer short periods of activity to longer stretches.

Everyone's health benefits when the whole family is involved in physical activity. Family activity also helps a child with weight issues feel a sense of family togetherness and lessens feelings of isolation. Older children are less likely to feel picked on if all family members are taking part in making a healthy-weight home.

The Von Dolteren Family Story

by Joanne Von Dolteren

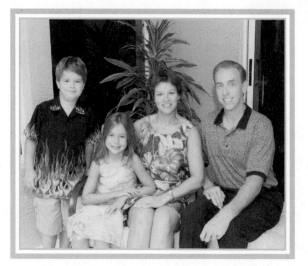

The Von Dolteren family spending quality time together

The only role model that my children know is the one who is in shape, takes exercise classes at the local Y, and runs in triathlons. My husband and I get some type of physical activity every day. The kids know that if we do not, we get cranky!

My young children do not know that I was not physically active as a child or that I struggled with my weight for most of my life. I didn't have a role model for activity. I am so pleased that my kids love being active as much as I do.

My children were just infants when I added daily activity to my life. I had lost weight after the birth of my second child, but my weight loss stalled with 25 pounds to go. I decided to help things along by getting a step-aerobics tape to watch at home. My husband and I got up each morning at 5:30 to exercise to the tape.

When a new Y opened in our area, we decided that physical activity should be a part of the kids' lives also. Our kids had us as role models; now they also had a place to go with activities just for kids, like indoor and outdoor playgrounds, a miniclimbing wall, and childcare that includes inside and outside playtime. While we take spinning and aerobics classes, the kids enjoy their own activities just for children.

They have so many choices: gym time, "kidsercise," running races, and even a step aerobics class just for kids.

The kids want to do the same activities we do. I love to run and so do the kids. Each year, our entire family runs in a local race that includes separate runs for adults and children. We look forward to being active together.

I fell in love with triathlons and had no idea that the kids were learning from watching me. I had just finished my first triathlon, with my husband and the kids on the sidelines rooting me on. A few weeks afterward, all of us were out by the pool. The kids didn't know how to swim yet, but they were doggie-paddling in the shallow end of the pool, then jumping out to ride their bikes, and then running in the yard. I couldn't figure out what they were doing. When I asked them to tell me about the game they were playing, they told me that they were in a triathlon!

I think that being a role model for activity has changed the course of my children's lives. My husband and I did not say anything to the children—we just did it and the kids followed our example.

Chapter 8

Putting Food
on the Table

As parents, we provide for our children. The basics are food, clothing, and shelter, but in today's world there is a whole lot more to being a provider. This chapter focuses on the role of the food provider. When it comes to food, the possibilities of what can be provided for meals and snacks are just about endless.

In creating a healthy-weight home, the goal is to provide both wholesome, nutritious foods and some treats. Being a food provider also means providing an atmosphere that is consistent in the way that the 5 Simple Rules are handled, being supportive about weight issues, and having an attitude that encourages healthy eating by the entire family. At the end of the chapter, you will meet the Davis family. A busy family of five, the Davises have made a lot of progress in the foods they provide for meals and snacks.

What Is a Food Provider?

Food providers do many important jobs. They are in charge of the family's eating schedule, that is, what time meals and snacks are served and where they are allowed to be eaten. They decide which foods to buy and how much to keep in the cupboards and refrigerator at home. It is

clearly the role of the parent, not the child, to decide what foods are
served at each meal.

Good Food Providers

- Establish regular meal and snack times
- Buy and prepare food
- Choose a fixed place for eating
- Are consistent in what foods are available
- Create a positive eating atmosphere
- Act as agents for change
- Maintain a positive attitude

Coach's Corner **Shopping for snacks**

Situation: One of the fathers was concerned about how his children would react if he limited the number of treats he buys on his weekly trip to the supermarket.

Strategies: I have often found that this concern is bigger in the mind of the parent than the reality of what happens when action is taken. My experience is that the vast majority of kids will eat healthy snacks without much fuss, especially if that is all that is available. They adjust pretty quickly to having only a limited number of treats available and understand that when they're gone, they're gone. Of course, giving a choice helps. I suggest to parents that they give children a choice of two foods, for example, a bowl of cereal or popcorn. By giving a set choice as opposed to asking "What would you like for a snack?" the stage is set for one of those foods to be selected. Dad tried this strategy and, lo and behold, it worked!

In making food choices for the family, the food provider limits how many treats are in the home. Limiting the number and types of treats that are brought into the house is an effective strategy, because it is hard to argue with a child about whether or not a food can be eaten if the food isn't there. For many of us, not having a lot of treats in the house also helps us to be better food role models.

All of us, adults and children alike, will find something we want to eat if we are really hungry. For example, a few whole-grain crackers with reduced-fat cheese can really hit the spot in the late afternoon. In addition, most children tend to be a little lazy and will eat whatever food is quick, easy, and available. If they find cookies, they will eat cookies—if they find yogurt, fresh fruits (the ultimate convenience food), and cut-up vegetables, that is what they will eat. A strategy that works for many families is to keep the wholesome foods at the front of the refrigerator and at eye level in the cupboards and store the treats in hard-to-reach places.

While not providing a lot of treats works, it is not recommended that all treats be banned from the house. Rather, a middle-of-the-road approach of buying a few treats makes sense. And while it may seem like a bargain, treats generally are not something that should be purchased in bulk. This makes sticking to Rule #2 easier.

Many of us think that if we simply do not provide any treats to our kids, they will learn not to want them. Unfortunately, this strategy usually backfires. Research finds that banning or putting extreme limits on treats tends to have the opposite effect on kids—children will like and want them more, not less. If the ban is strictly enforced, children are also likely to sneak the food into the house. The last thing any of us wants to do is help create a closet eater.

Just as with being a food role model, it's best to make small, gradual changes in the ways food is provided to the family. Little changes are easier for all family members, kids and adults alike, to adjust to. Small steps do add up, especially with children. Tried and true steps for families to begin with include switching from oil to a cooking spray for sautéing; going down one level of fat percentage in milk (e.g., from whole milk to 2% or 1% to nonfat); serving only low-fat or nonfat milk or water as a beverage with meals; buying extra lean groundmeat (at least 93% fat-free); switching from refined grains to whole grains; buying more fruit; and making a salad a routine side dish at dinner.

It is easier to be a food provider when the food is eaten at home. After all, what is bought at the grocery store is what is available to eat. The role of the food provider becomes more difficult when the family is eating out, because the provider is giving the money to pay for the food rather than providing the food itself. A restaurant offers a variety of menu items and family members provide for themselves. The provider does have a say about what restaurant will be chosen and so can pick places that have more wholesome food choices available. That said, many of us find that making the choice to eat more simple meals at home and fewer meals out is what works best.

Parents create a healthy-weight home by buying and cooking wholesome, nutritious foods and preparing meals that help kids make wise food choices. They also provide beverage choices that do not have a lot of calories.

In the role of the food provider, parents allow children to decide how much food they want to eat to match their feelings of hunger and fullness. Doing this promotes the practice of children eating only when they truly are hungry and stopping when full. By asking questions about hunger and fullness and then giving food in response to those answers, parents play a central role in teaching children to eat only what their body needs to grow and develop. This strategy does not take a lot of time or effort. Simply asking a child who has come home from school "Are you hungry for a snack?" helps to reveal what is truly going on with the child's hunger rather than just assuming that an after-school snack is needed out of habit.

As parents, we learn to find the right balance between keeping regular meal and snack times and allowing enough flexibility to respond to feelings of hunger. A consistent enforcement of the boundaries, regardless of what they are, provides kids with the structure they want and need.

Coach's Corner Recognizing hunger

Situation: A mother understood the need to encourage her daughter to eat before getting too hungry, but at the same time she did not want unplanned snacks to ruin her child's appetite for dinner.

Strategies: One of the biggest challenges for me is helping parents figure out if their kids are truly hungry. The first step for this mother was to help her daughter learn the difference between true hunger and the urge to eat for other reasons, like boredom, fatigue, or frustration. She did this by asking questions. If the child was not really hungry, they talked about what had made her want to eat and found nonfood activities that would fill the void. If the daughter was truly hungry, they talked about how intense the hunger was. If the hunger was intense, she gave her a small snack. If the feeling was rated as medium and dinner was not too far off, she encouraged her daughter to wait. This strategy began to work over time because it helped the daughter think about feelings of hunger and learn that getting hungry before a meal is good because it means that the level of hunger will be just about right when it is time for dinner.

We food providers set up policies that affect everyone who lives in the home. For example, we may decide that food can only be eaten in the kitchen and the dining room, that dinners are not served with the television on, and that salad is served with dinner every night—a great way to cut down on calories. Over time and with consistency, the foods that are provided become the fabric of the way our family eats and are part of the daily food routine. To the family members who live in the home, exceptions to the food policies become abnormal and undesirable.

> ### Coach's Corner   **Managing treats**
>
> **Situation:** I was talking to a mother and father about the weight-loss program they recently joined. They told me that in an effort to cut calories, they stocked the pantry with lots of their usual treats, but bought them in lower-calorie, lower-sugar, or lower-fat versions. Soon, the whole family was eating a lot of reduced-fat cookies and light ice cream. While they were cutting calories, they thought that they might not be providing the kinds of foods that the family should really be focusing on.
>
> **Strategies:** I wish that more parents would make better choices by switching away from full-fat and sugary treats. However, so many people I know simply keep too many treats in the house. If the treats are there, most of us will eat them too often. Once we discussed this, Mom and Dad decided to cut down on the number of treats that they were buying and started buying more wholesome foods, like fruits, low-fat dairy foods, and whole-grain crackers and cereals, to eat as snacks.

We parents have the ability to introduce new foods to our families. In this role, we take advantage of the opportunity to expose kids to new foods, like asparagus, artichokes, or mango. Plus, we are able to expose our children to new restaurant experiences, like a sushi bar or a vegetarian restaurant. Expanding the horizons of healthy food options is a great strategy because it helps the entire family to enjoy the fun of eating without giving up the basics of having a healthy-weight home.

Infants

Infants rely entirely on their providers for all their food needs. Shortly after giving birth, new moms decide whether to breast-feed or bottle feed. There is strong scientific support behind the advantages of breast-feeding: it boosts the baby's immune system, provides nutrients for brain development, and appears to be linked with a lower risk of excess weight in childhood. Breast-feeding can also help a mother to return to her prepregnancy weight. Because nursing allows babies to control how much milk they take, they are more likely to match their intake with the calories they need.

While there are benefits to nursing, it is not the right choice for every mother or every baby. Bottle feeding (using pumped breast milk or formula) is a perfectly fine way to feed infants, and bottle-fed babies grow and develop normally.

What works for infants is to listen and watch carefully for their signals—they know when they want to eat and when they want to stop. Responding to these cues both before and toward the end of a feeding helps children fine-tune the natural senses of hunger and fullness they were born with. This practice applies to both breast-fed and bottle-fed babies. Those taking a bottle should have it taken away with the first signs of being full, whether the bottle is empty or not.

First foods for babies should be introduced in very, very small portions. As with bottle feeding or breast-feeding, paying close attention to a baby's signals for hunger and fullness is helpful. Infancy is the perfect time for babies to try a variety of different vegetables. Many experts recommend buying baby foods that do not have added sugar, fat, or starch.

What doesn't work is feeding a baby without learning the baby's different cues for hunger and fullness, reactions to new flavors and textures, and feelings of discomfort. Babies often frown and make faces when they are given a new food. They may also refuse or spit out new foods. This is natural and should not be seen as a rejection of the food—for now or for life. Experts recommend that babies be given the same new food at several meals in a row. It generally takes between ten and fourteen times for a baby to accept a new food.

Toddlers and Young Children

Toddlers and young children rely on their parents not only to buy their food but also to get it on the plate. At this stage of a child's development, the challenge has as much to do with feeding behavior as it does with nutrition. One of the best ways for toddlers and young children to state their desire for independence is by making food demands. To eat or not to eat is one of the few things a young child has control over.

What works for toddlers and young children is to keep emotions out of eating. If a child cannot get a reaction, the behavior is usually abandoned. The best strategy for working with a child who is fussy, picky, or cranky is to show no reaction at all when it comes to food.

Children tend to be more positive about trying new foods when they are calm and not afraid of tasting something new. Providing a quiet mealtime environment helps a young child feel relaxed. It also helps to give a new food to the whole family—with strict instructions that there are to be no negative words or body language to make the young child think that the food is yucky. Doing this helps remove some of the young child's natural fear factor. It is common for young kids to be fickle with food—to like certain foods one day and not the next. For this reason, it helps to keep providing a food that was initially not liked to take advantage of this childhood trait. Many of us have the mistaken belief that our child hates a food simply because we provided it once and it was rejected. With time, exposure, and an expanded palate, young children are likely to like the vast majority of foods we give them.

Coach's Corner　　**War against vegetables**

Situation: A mother came to me with a familiar problem: her young son would not eat vegetables and she was tired of fighting over broccoli every night. She worried about whether he was getting all the nutrition that he needed.

Strategies: Many parents are surprised when I point out that fruits supply many of the same nutrients and health benefits of vegetables. Her son loved fruit. Knowing this, she decided that she would put a bowl of grapes on the table at dinner instead of putting the dreaded broccoli on his plate. He ate the grapes and, to Mom's delight, the mealtime stress level was low. For now, Mom's strategy is to focus on providing more fruits. With time, however, she hopes to make another round with the vegetables—though not broccoli.

Many of us find the idea of letting kids decide how much to eat a challenge. It is a challenge worth overcoming, though, because it is one of the steps that puts children on the path to a healthy weight. Research shows that preschool children have a fairly steady calorie intake when they are allowed to listen and respond to their own hunger and fullness signals. Encouraging children to decide how much to eat helps them to balance the calories they are eating with the calories their body needs at that time. The focus on wholesome, nutritious foods in a healthy-weight home makes it less likely that children will overeat. If excess weight is already an issue, parents can try starting off with smaller first portions, then providing more if requested; encouraging the child to eat more slowly; and providing a lot of vegetables, fruit, broth-based soups, salads, and other filling foods that have a lot of water but not a lot of calories.

Coach's Corner **The big eater**

Situation: I was approached by a mother and father whose toddler always had a big appetite from the time that he was a baby. They didn't want him to be hungry but were afraid he was overeating. Without guidance, they said, he could eat the family out of house and home.

Strategies: This challenge needed a few different healthy-weight strategies. We discussed that as providers, they should help their son take appropriate-sized portions and serve him only small amounts if he asked for seconds. They learned to watch him for signs that he was getting full even if his eating was not slowing down, and to ask him periodically about his feelings of fullness. To end meals without a fight, they encouraged him to be excused to play, offering to save his leftovers in case he got hungry later.

Young children can be gently guided toward eating suitable portions. Questions about fullness—"Does your tummy feel really full?" or "Does your tummy feel empty?"—prompts a young child to stop eating for a moment and think about hunger levels.

All ethnic heritages and cultures include wholesome, nutritious foods, making the 5 Simple Rules doable for every household. There is no need to abandon food traditions to provide a healthy-weight home.

Coach's Corner   Ethnic cuisine

Situation: A mother of five told me that she believed that the foods from her country were not healthy. Rice and beans were the foundation of her diet growing up and also of the diet of her family.

Strategies: Mom was genuinely surprised when I told her that just a few simple changes could make her favorite dishes more wholesome and nutritious. The first change she made was changing white rice to brown in the family's rice and beans recipe. The kids did not notice, and because her husband supported her efforts, he did not say anything either. She found that the kids ate less because the brown rice was more filling than white. We agreed that she could also work on introducing more vegetables and fruits, including her traditional ones like peppers, onions, and plantains. She began cooking with less oil, another change that went unnoticed by her family. As she told me after making many changes, "Like all children, my kids love their Mom's cooking."

While focusing on wholesome, nutritious foods is important, so is including treats. When children are provided with treats that are their personal favorites, they feel empowered, are more satisfied, and get extra pleasure from the treat because it was their choice.

What doesn't work is encouraging children to continue eating when they are no longer hungry. The challenge is to find out if the child is full or just distracted and not paying attention to eating. Children who stop eating after a few bites or skip a meal completely need a gentle reminder that food will not be served until the next snack or meal. If they do not continue after the reminder, that is okay and the meal should be stopped. However, the child should not be fed again until the next regular meal or snack. Children will not starve by missing a meal or two and the lessons learned by having a few missed meals are valuable. Reacting to a missed or refused meal by providing different foods and giving in to a child's demands weakens our ability to have a healthy-weight home.

Many kids have a built-in preference for foods that are high in fat and calories. Because the calories in these foods are highly concentrated, high-fat foods are easy to overeat. These foods need to be designated as treats and provided in accordance with Rule #2.

Just as catering to a child's food preferences is not helpful, neither is using food as a reward. To a child, getting a food reward, especially if it is a treat, makes that food seem more special and it may become highly desirable.

Parents should give both familiar and new foods to the family with very little fuss. Toddlers and young children tend to accept the foods they are provided as long as they have no reason to suspect that the foods are different. Calling attention to a food swap, for example, replacing 1% milk with fat-free milk, can cause a child to reject the new milk.

(*Coach's Corner*)　　**Juice swap**

Situation: At the end of a discussion about limiting juice, a mother of two young girls admitted to me that she was giving them juice in amounts that far exceeded the recommended half-cup per day. She did not know what to give them as an alternative, because she believed they would not accept water as a substitute.

Strategies: Since young children often can't tell if juice has been diluted, Mom diluted their usual apple juice with water to make it less concentrated. Her girls did not notice the difference. In her efforts to create a healthy-weight home, she also switched from full-fat dairy products to 2% cheese and low-fat frozen yogurt. Again, her daughters did not notice. Her success was exactly what I expected!

Older Children

Older children are both easier and harder than younger children. Older children are able to understand how their food choices affect their weight. However, as a form of adolescent rebellion, older children may not want to follow the 5 Simple Rules. Experts recommend that parents in these circumstances continue to provide wholesome, nutritious meals to older children, even if their efforts seem to be undermined by the child eating out, bringing extra treats into the house, or missing meals. It's important to have a strong belief that you are doing the right thing. Often the lessons that are learned as a young child and rejected as a teen return in young adulthood.

What works for older children is to keep introducing new foods to the family. As kids enter their preteen years, they may be more willing to try new foods, even if some of the new foods do not taste good to them. This is different from what is seen with younger children, who react to one unliked new food with an unwillingness to try any other new food.

Older children often invade the kitchen, eating whatever is easy, tasty, and available. Stocking up on wholesome foods is an effective strategy. Research shows that when these foods are provided and ready to eat, kids will eat more of them. In addition, not providing sugar-containing soft drinks and fruit juices limits the amount that an older child will drink. This is a particularly good strategy because these beverages have been linked to a higher BMI and increased chances of weight gain.

Parents aid sensible eating habits by serving an appropriate number of foods in the proper portion sizes. Food package labels offer portion guidance—you may be surprised to learn that a single packaged muffin, for example, counts as two or even three servings. Portion control is particularly important for treats.

Coach's Corner | America's favorite eating holiday

Situation: Just before Thanksgiving, parents often talk to me about the challenge of creating a healthy-weight home during a holiday that is all about eating large amounts of food. A father of two children was particularly concerned about what to do.

Strategies: We discussed cutting down on the number of dishes and limiting them to those traditional foods that his family members really enjoyed. He chose to prepare a turkey, fresh vegetables, stuffing, and just one type of pie, pumpkin. He left out the mashed potatoes, rolls, and pecan pie. Everyone had a nice meal and nobody commented about the foods that were missing. When I saw him the next week, he was amazed.

Food providers can help avoid potentially tough situations. For example, if the school cafeteria does not provide healthful choices or the child does not select them, we can pack a brown bag lunch. If asked why, a simple statement about a need to save money as the reason is usually accepted.

(Coach's Corner)   Avoiding the avoidable

Situation: After seeing a documentary on super-sized portions that included a look at school lunches, a mother told me how concerned she was about what her daughter was eating in school. She was not sure how to provide a better lunch for her.

Strategies: One of the first steps was for Mom to find out exactly what foods were available at school. She arranged to eat lunch at school with her daughter and was upset by the quality and portion size of school cafeteria food. Although having her daughter buy lunch was easier, she decided to send lunch from home.

What doesn't work is strict food restrictions. Children who are not allowed to eat when they are truly hungry get the message that they should eat when food is around instead of when they are hungry. This does not mean, however, that food should be given freely when a child refuses or misses a meal by his or her own choice. True hunger takes many hours to develop and the likelihood of harmful hunger taking place between the meals and snacks provided in the typical home is almost nil.

In addition, extreme food rules may cause children to eat more when they are not hungry. Research finds that mothers who restrict their own eating and also experience periods when they are out of control around food tend to restrict their daughters, who are then more prone to overeat and gain weight as a result.

Being overly authoritarian in our role as food providers lessens the chances of creating a healthy-weight home. Children respond best to providers who are consistent, firm, and supportive.

Finally, it is important to be consistent food providers for everyone in the family. When children with excess weight are given different foods and different rules from those for their lean siblings, confidence and self-esteem are affected and feelings of deprivation are more likely. That is one of the big reasons why the 5 Simple Rules apply to everyone.

Coach's Corner   **All in the family**

Situation: A mother and father with one overweight daughter and one in the healthy-weight range wanted advice on buying foods and serving meals just for the daughter facing weight challenges.

Strategies: We discussed the likely poor results of following this strategy, something they had never considered. Mom and Dad realized that their daughter would be more successful and they would be healthier if the entire family ate the same foods. They switched to fat-free milk and both daughters pack their lunch for school. Dad even started drinking water with his meals, something he never did in the past.

The Davis Family Story

by Anica Davis

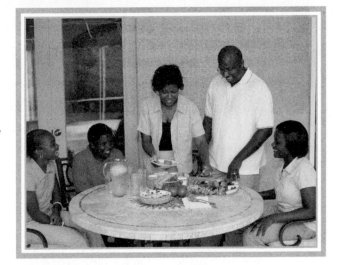

The Davis family getting ready to eat

Providing food for our three teenagers is a challenge. We're a very busy family. Often our choice is between eating on the run and having dinner after nine in the evening once our kids get home from their extracurricular activities. But my husband and I knew that if we didn't provide wholesome, nutritious foods to our kids they might never learn about healthy eating.

My husband and I had changed the way that we ate because we were trying to lose weight. We were so motivated by our success that we decided to feed our kids in a similar way. The kids quickly learned that meals at home were a priority and that it was important to find time to fit family meals into our hectic schedules.

The kids are teenagers, so they were old enough to sit down together to discuss ways that we could change our family eating habits. We planned family menus by choosing recipes from cookbooks and then making a grocery list for me to shop with. The kids will eat almost anything, so we try many different types of dishes. They enjoy foods that they did not eat before, like fish—we bread it with a cornflake crust and bake it in the oven—and shrimp. It would have been all too easy to fall into the trap of cooking only what is familiar and quick. Some things haven't worked very well, like trying to switch to whole wheat bread. My kids just won't eat bread that is brown.

As a food provider, I have become a more careful label reader. I always bought ground turkey for burgers but never read the labels before. It turns out that the store brand I was buying was just as high in fat as regular ground beef. Now I only buy lower-fat ground turkey.

We have a list of wholesome foods that are in the house all of the time. When the kids want a snack, they have plenty of foods to choose from. I still have cookies in the house, but our choices have changed to healthier varieties and we eat them only as treats. Planning our foods and meals together works better than if I were forcing the kids to eat certain things.

Our kitchen is filled with fruits and vegetables. In the past, I couldn't pay my son to eat green beans. Now he loves them. He has taken ownership of his fruit eating—if he does not have fruit at breakfast, he packs a piece to take for lunch. Nectarines have replaced rice cereal bars as his favorite dessert! My other kids also are big vegetable lovers. Broccoli is a favorite, along with baby carrots dipped in fat-free ranch dressing.

We have made so many changes in the way we eat: reduced-fat popcorn as a snack (the kids used to make fun of me for eating it), plenty of water and much less fruit juice, different types of fruits and vegetables, and lots of fish. I know that we are not perfect but I don't worry about it. The changes we have made in the foods we eat are huge!

Chapter 9

Helping Kids Move

How can a parent provide activity? This chapter takes a look at the many ways that we can be activity providers. You will also meet the Neeley family. This family of four decided to tackle activity head on and is finding that they are having a lot of fun.

What Is an Activity Provider?

For many children, the best way to provide activity is to make sure that they have plenty of opportunities to be active. Children have naturally high levels of energy, a fact that is often envied by adults. Kids love to run around playing and having fun. Outdoor games are an endless source of entertainment. Many of us think back fondly to our childhood days when we had so much energy.

Most children, given the chance, will be active on their own. Sometimes kids need a little help, though, to spark their natural instincts. Activity providers light the spark by providing toys and sports equipment, giving rides to classes and games, inviting other kids to come to the house to play, and reminding kids of the fun that they can have playing outside.

In today's world, kids often need equipment to enjoy their chosen activities. The activity provider makes sure that the equipment is available. The kinds of equipment a child may need are easy: Frisbees,

> **Good Activity Providers**
>
> - Buy sports equipment and toys
> - Provide emotional actions:
>   Support
>   Encouragement
>   Praise
>   Motivation
>   Feedback
>   Reinforcement

balls, riding toys, bicycles, footballs, in-line skates, and anything else that a game requires. Also on the list are car rides, registration fees, and the time that it takes to attend practices or games. Activity providers can take an extra step by volunteering to be coaches, assistants, and referees.

Coach's Corner   Activities for all seasons

Situation: The parents of two girls, a young girl and a preteen, talked to me about how their family could become more active. They needed help with ideas that the whole family could enjoy year round, both at home and when visiting the grandparents in Michigan.

Strategies: We came up with a lot of different options that the family could do wherever they were. During the school year, the girls could play outside right after school before it got dark. The family could walk to the community pool in the summer and to the local sledding hills when they were in Michigan. A walk around the neighborhood could be anywhere, anytime. With this in mind, an after-dinner family walk became part of their daily routine. They also all got scooters to ride on their street. In addition, Mom found that she enjoyed walking with the girls to the local playground and playing with them on the equipment.

Families have options when it comes to activity, including both unstructured activities like playing and bike riding and organized activities like team sports. Structured activities often require adjustments in the family schedule to make room for the lessons, practices, and games that are part of organized sports. Within the family, activity providers give encouragement and support to their kids by being cheerleaders. Praising a child's efforts can be a strong motivator for a child to stay active. Many children are reluctant to try an activity without a gentle push from behind. Showing interest and recognizing achievements when progress is made, being empathetic when things do not go so well, and offering useful suggestions for improvement are all part of being an activity provider. This is especially important during the not-so-fun times because it helps a child stick with it.

Research finds that parents' belief in their child's ability to perform pays off—children whose parents believe in them are more likely to join an activity that is physically challenging. Confidence in children's abilities and support for their choice to play a sport fosters children who are confident about their physical skills, have a good attitude, are motivated, and participate more often.

The activity provider creates a healthy-weight home by encouraging and making daily activity possible. Regular activity is so important that it is one of the 5 Simple Rules. A home environment that is committed to activity helps inspire the kids to want to be active.

Having fun as the primary goal of activity makes it more likely that children will want to be part of the action. Experts agree that young children should not be forced to exercise as a means to lose weight, and many adolescents will not exercise simply to lose or maintain weight. Except for the unusually motivated child, activity quickly can become drudgery if it is missing the fun factor. In a healthy-weight home, activities are enjoyable, rewarding, and in sync with the family's lifestyle. The health and weight benefits are a bonus.

Children enjoy activities when adults provide support and are involved themselves. Children love to hear compliments from adults.

Kids Enjoy Activity When They

- Have parents who are supportive and involved
- Receive compliments
- Feel confident in their own ability
- Try new skills
- Master new skills
- Experience the joy of movement

The fun factor of activity goes up when children are confident of their abilities—throwing and catching a ball, running, jumping, and swimming. Parents can help by giving children a challenge that stretches their abilities and helps them to learn and master new physical skills. Activity is more fun when there is a challenge to conquer. Children also love the feeling of movement, like the wind in their faces when riding a bicycle, the sensation of speed in their legs while skating, and the rush of water over their body during swimming. Taking the time to build fun into activity helps children develop a lifelong love of movement.

In creating a healthy-weight home, a balance between two of the 5 Simple Rules needs to be created: including at least sixty minutes daily of physical activity and limiting screen time to two hours or less a day. Since most kids get only thirty minutes or so of activity each day, that means aiming to add an additional thirty minutes. Where does this come from? The most effective strategy for most families is to cut back on screen time and other types of sedentary time.

Research shows that creating an atmosphere that boosts the child's "can do" confidence helps the child master his or her favorite skills and encourages goal setting to learn new skills. Confident kids are more likely to be happy, motivated, and active. This type of home environment also nurtures children who are more likely to take part in physical activity and enjoy it more.

Action Plans for Providing Activity

Family activities for exercise and enjoyment

Opportunities for children to participate in household activities like walking the dog, washing the car, or working in the garden

A safe environment for children and their friends to play and enjoy physical activities such as swimming, biking, skating, and ball sports

Encouragement to try or continue a new activity

A way to get there

Equipment, uniforms, and necessary gear

Alternatives to screen time and other sedentary activities

Infants

Every infant needs activity providers. Infants cannot move very far on their own, so they rely on parents and caregivers to take them from the crib to the play area. They need playtime to move their arms and legs, to practice reaching and grabbing, and to get help standing, bouncing, and learning to move on their own. Blocks, stuffed animals, and other toys that encourage babies to play are the responsibility of the activity provider. When buying toys, it is a good strategy to think in terms of whether the toy will help the baby move.

What works for infants is getting at least an hour of active playtime every day. Most babies cannot play for an hour straight. Instead, a better strategy is to work in blocks of time when babies can play with family members and explore their small world. Babies need an interesting and safe place to play, creep, and crawl, for example, a large blanket or mat on the floor.

What doesn't work is long periods in a crib, infant seat, play pen, or stroller. Young infants who sit or lie down for long periods of time are not likely to get enough activity.

Toddlers and Young Children

Being an activity provider for a toddler or young child can be hard work! In fact, most parents with kids this age say that the kids are the activity providers for them. Young children need constant companionship and supervision as they move around at breakneck speed. Their interests and skills change quickly, so it is important to be on the ball with new and more challenging activities.

What works for young children is providing lots of outside playtime. Research finds that kids who play outside are more active overall. The other benefit of playing outside is that it keeps kids away from the attractions of being inside, like televisions, computers, and video games.

Young kids need a time and place to be active. Given the opportunity, most children will jump right in. Research shows that children will choose to play, as long as they have the chance to learn and practice new skills and receive praise. Children's enthusiasm can be encouraged even more by helping them to master different skills.

Physical activity is more than playing, joining a team sport, or exercising. An easy way to get a child more active is to work movement into his or her daily routines. Where feasible, a terrific strategy is to walk rather than drive to school. A daily family dog walk is a winner for everyone—adults, kids, and the dog. Nearby errands can be done on foot or by bike instead of in the car. At the market or mall, the car can be parked at the furthest parking space rather than the closest one and the stroller can be left in the car. The young child's only option is to walk.

Coach's Corner   **Changing a mindset**

Situation: A mother of two young girls wanted them to be more active. But after a long day at work, she was too tired to go outside and play with them after dinner. She wanted to know if I had any suggestions.

Strategies: As soon as we started talking, Mom realized that what she really needed to change was her own beliefs about activity. So instead of making a heroic effort to plan activities in her few free hours after dinner, she decided to combine physical activity with those events that were already part of the family's daily routine. For example, she and her daughters walked rather than drove to the local duck pond for their weekly trip to feed the ducks. They also walked over a mile to visit the girls' grandfather on Sundays, who then drove them home.

Providing activities can be simply moving, like taking an afternoon walk in the park, walking around the mall, or spending some time at a local playground. Another effective strategy is to invite a child's friend to come over and play outside for a few hours. It helps to try to have at least a few kids in a child's circle of playmates who enjoy being active.

Early childhood is the best time to build a child's self-esteem about being active. Research shows that parents who show confidence in their child's ability to do an activity help increase the child's motivation to continue with the activity. Most young children are not yet ready to benefit from competitive sports. Activities that provide the greatest boost to a young child's self-esteem are those that reward participation and effort rather than winning. Examples include swimming lessons and dance classes.

Coach's Corner Options for young children

Situation: During a discussion on being an activity provider, a mother mentioned that she wanted to offer her two preschoolers more opportunities to be active. She was looking for options that could help her children build the physical skills that they would need when they got older and that could help build their confidence.

Strategies: I recommended that she seek out information about activity options that are available in the community. For example, I knew that a Y in this mother's community offered a wide range of afternoon activities for young children. Learning this, she signed her kids up for a membership and enrolled them in an afternoon program with different activities every day. One day of the week the children go outside to play games. On another day, their activity was an exercise with simple movements that preschoolers could master. The Y also had large and small balls and other movement toys for children to play with under supervision. The kids love it.

As parents, many of us are surprised to find that our kids actually prefer being active over being sedentary. Often, children watch television or play on the computer out of boredom—they cannot think of other things to do on their own. Once they have been provided with interesting alternatives, they realize how much more fun it is to be active than to sit inside.

Coach's Corner   Neighborhood fun

Situation: A group of us were discussing how much we loved going outside and playing with other kids in the neighborhood when we were young. One of the mothers wanted to try to create the same experience for her children.

Strategies: We all agreed that kickball was a simple outdoor game that her children could master easily and enjoy playing. She suggested to her kids that she teach them how to play kickball in the front yard where the neighbors could see them playing. It was very fun. As the expression from the movie *Field of Dreams* goes, "If you build it, they will come." Within a matter of weeks, the neighbors started joining in, and kickball is now the neighborhood's after-dinner activity of choice.

What doesn't work is emphasizing activity only for the child or children with weight issues. Physical activity is more fun when everyone in the family takes part. Encouraging just the heavy child to be more active can make activity feel like a punishment for being overweight. When everyone else gets to stay home, watching television or playing on the computer, the child who is pushed into being active can feel excluded. As a result, television watching and playing on the computer will become even more attractive.

Encouraging one child who has natural athletic ability and not encouraging another who is less coordinated can make activity less enjoyable to the less athletic child. In one study, parents gave more encouragement to their sons than to their daughters. The researchers found that the daughters felt less capable and lacked enthusiasm about being active.

Coach's Corner — Activity options

Situation: A mother and father were very active physically—they played softball in a coed softball league, basketball, and doubles tennis. They could not understand why, when they were so active themselves, their preteen son's activity of choice was to spend time at home on his computer.

Strategies: We talked about not forcing their son to play an organized sport. Just because that was the way they enjoyed being active doesn't mean that their son would enjoy that also. I told them that forcing him to play a sport that he didn't enjoy or didn't have the confidence to play could turn him off to the idea of activity altogether. However, we agreed that it was reasonable to require their son to participate in some kind of after-school activity to get him out of the house and away from his computer. They did some research and found out about cooking classes for kids, music classes, and scout meetings, which were all in line with his interests. He signed up for scouting and discovered that he enjoyed spending time outdoors with other kids.

It is not enough just to be an activity role model. Children are not automatically active just because the adults around them are. Kids also need activity providers who give them the opportunities and encouragement to be active.

Given the reality of today's world, we cannot leave it up to the schools to make sure that our children get the amount of activity they need. Budget cuts and an increased focus on academics have caused many districts to eliminate physical education, recess, and competitive and recreational sports. Furthermore, those schools that have made a concerted effort to make their elementary-age students more active have had mixed results. Forced activity, whether on the individual or the school level, has a tendency to backfire. While schools can help, they cannot be the primary providers of physical activity.

Older Children

Older children have different motivations for being active. They have already mastered the basic physical skills—jumping, running, throwing, and climbing—and are ready to advance to new skills. Older children are keenly aware of competition and accomplishment. They know which kids are the fastest, strongest, and best athletes. As children get older, friends become a bigger motivation for activity than parents. The role of activity provider changes somewhat during these years, but it remains important.

What works for older children is lots of support for their chosen activities. The activity provider helps children be physically active by signing them up for sports teams, driving to practices, helping arrange active playdates, and providing whatever the children need in the way of uniforms and equipment to participate. Through their support, kids get the message that physical activity is important.

(Coach's Corner)   **Exploring what's available**

Situation: The mother of a preteen asked for help in providing activity options for her son. He was highly motivated to step up his activity level but was not interested in trying out for a sports team and was not yet in shape to join a structured program.

Strategies: We explored a variety of options, including a youth membership at a local fitness center, an exercise class for pre-teens, or a couple of sessions with a personal trainer who could teach him exercises to do on his own. Mom also started to look for activities for the entire family, like bicycling and walking. With several choices to pick from, Mom was sure that her son would find an activity or activities that appealed to him.

Older children thrive on positive feedback and encouragement, whether it is from their parents, siblings, or peers. Research finds that getting support from parents and peers motivates older children to be more active. Children in general and girls in particular are also more active when they believe that parents are backing them up.

In addition, the competitive streak in older children is a strong motivator. They like chances to compete against their friends as a way to measure and show off their abilities. For those older children who enjoy competition, encouraging them to challenge themselves and others works. This may mean joining a team sport, challenging friends to a game of basketball, or working toward a personal best in resistance training or running.

As with younger children, decreasing inactivity by limiting screen time is a good strategy for older kids. Between prime-time television shows, homework, e-mail, instant messaging, and video games, older children have too many opportunities for screen time. Several studies find that children who spend the most time in front of a screen are most likely to face weight challenges: over half of the excess weight gain in older children is linked to too much screen time.

> **Coach's Corner**　　　**Balancing screen time**
>
> **Situation:** One of the mothers realized that her family watched way too much television, so she wanted to cut down on everyone's screen time, but her son, who played sports and had gym class at the middle school he attended, liked to use the television to relax after an active day at school and several hours of homework. Mom felt bad trying to enforce the rule that limits screen time since he already was so active.
>
> **Strategies:** It can be a tough situation to handle when one family member already is very active. However, we discussed the importance of being consistent in applying the 5 Simple Rules so that nobody would feel singled out or punished. By enforcing limits on the family's screen time, Mom was pleasantly surprised to find how easily her son came up with other ways to relax, including listening to music and reading sports magazines.

What doesn't work for older children is forcing family time. Older children enjoy spending time with friends—to many, being with their parents is just not cool. Older children may rebel if they are pushed too hard to participate in family activities. At this age, being a role model for activity is no longer a guarantee that the child will be active. Older children need to be provided with activities that they will enjoy, especially if they can be done with friends.

> **Coach's Corner**　　　**The reluctant teen**
>
> **Situation:** Despite numerous attempts to do activities as a family, a couple was discouraged because their teenage daughter was going through the stage of not wanting to spend time with them. They tried to provide other opportunities for her to be more active, but nothing appealed to her.

Strategies: One strategy that works is to make teenagers come up with their own ideas, making clear that not having any ideas is not an option. In this case, their daughter said that she would take walks as long as she could walk by herself. They gave the okay as long as she walked with the dog, a strategy that was a win-win for the teen and the dog.

While it is true for younger children, it is even truer that older children are unlikely to get recommended levels of activity as part of their school day. Many schools offer limited opportunity for activity and some allow students to go through an entire school year without participating in any kind of physical activity. As parents, we can provide the opportunities for our children to be active, and if we want or need a next step, we can become advocates (discussed in chapter 13) with the schools to provide more opportunities there.

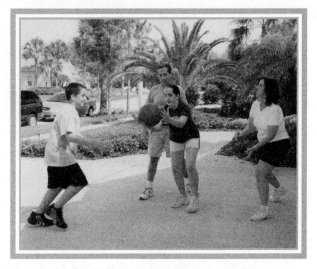

The Neeley family likes to shoot hoops together

The Neeley Family Story

by Debbie Neeley

Ken and I didn't think much about activity for our family. We had not been very active as a family—no family walks, bike rides, or outdoor games together. Then one day our pediatrician told us that our two adolescent kids' BMIs were slightly higher than they should be. At that moment, we knew that we needed to do something for the entire family.

Since both of us struggle with our weight, we wanted to help our children avoid the same challenges. Healthy eating was already a part of our lives, so we knew that providing family activities would be a big help.

Our goal was to get the kids enthusiastic about family activities. Convincing adolescents to be more active is not always easy. First, we suggested to our children that all of us run or bicycle together since Ken and I enjoy doing both. The kids were not very interested. The quick lesson we learned was that kids may not enjoy what their parents do.

We tried a different strategy and asked other parents what types of activities their kids enjoyed. One parent mentioned Dance Dance Revolution, a video game that has kids copy dance moves. We bought the game and our children love it. Another new favorite is Twister

Moves. The great thing about these games is that the kids think they are playing a game; in the meantime, they are raising their heart rate and getting physical activity.

With our encouragement, the kids gradually have become more active. Our son plays a lot of sports—baseball, football, basketball, and tennis—but did not do much between seasons. Now when his dad asks him to go jogging, he says yes once in a while. The two of them ran in a Thanksgiving morning 5K Turkey Trot; our daughter and I walked the course. It was great to burn off calories before we even started the day. Our daughter is more active than she used to be. We found a low-key, noncompetitive sports league for her so that she can feel successful without a lot of stress. She also horseback rides, an activity she truly enjoys. Our goal is to keep finding activities she likes to do.

Our kids have seen positive results and are more motivated to be active now. The key factor is for parents to play two roles: provider and role model. As providers, we enabled our children to participate. As role models, we changed things in our own lives, not just in the lives of our children.

Physical activity has to be a family thing, with parents as leaders.

Chapter 10

Setting Food Policy

So far we have discussed two of the five roles that we as parents play in making a healthy-weight home. Now it is time to move on to the role of enforcer. As with being a role model and provider, the role of enforcer is so important that the food and activity aspects are covered separately. This chapter deals with food, and chapter 11 explores activity. While the term "enforcer" may sound harsh, the role of being a food enforcer does not need to be, as you will see when you read about the Beal family at the end of this chapter.

What Is a Food Enforcer?

As parents, we set the rules of the house, everything from whether or not beds need to be made every morning to what beverage will be served with meals. We are the enforcers of the family. Being an effective enforcer can be a particularly challenging role because it requires a fine balance between imposing the rules too strictly and not being tough enough.

Children need structure, and nowhere is this truer than in their family life. Kids need structure because it provides the framework they use to build their lives. The structure children use to build their lives is like a house—it needs a strong foundation and solid walls to last. Once the building is done, children can decorate their house to match their personalities and style.

While children want and need structure, they also need flexibility. How much depends on how old they are, with more needed as they grow from being babies to young adults. While it would be terrific if the whole growing up process went smoothly, it rarely does. Children fight against the rules of the house as a way to gain more flexibility. This is not uncommon. Just as it is our job to enforce the rules, it is the child's job to protest them.

Good Food Enforcers

- Agree about what the rules are and their priority
- Are consistent but not rigid
- Create the family food environment
- Support positive influences
- Promote healthy food choices
- Support the family's food and eating behaviors
- Counteract negative influences

In creating a healthy-weight home, the food enforcer makes the family eating policies stick. In addition, a child's food choices and eating patterns are profoundly affected by the food enforcer. One example is helping kids learn to listen to their body's signals of hunger and fullness and then providing food to match the signals. If a child is not hungry but wants to eat out of boredom, the food enforcer does not provide a snack, because *we do not eat if we are not truly hungry*. However, if a child is truly hungry, food is provided. These actions of enforcement—food for hunger, not for boredom—back up and reinforce the role model and provider roles when it comes to dealing with food.

On a more basic level, we parents decide how the 5 Simple Rules will work in our family. We are the ones who create the boundaries and, more important, are consistent in enforcing the boundaries we have created. We decide what time meals and snacks are served, which foods are treats, and what beverages are allowed with meals. The goal of this role is not to be a food cop but to make sure that when it comes to food and eating, the family is doing things that promote health, well-being, and a healthy weight. The role of food enforcer focuses on those foods and eating behaviors that affect the whole family.

Many of us find the encouraging rules—like eating more wholesome, nutritious foods and being more active—easier to enforce. It is often harder to find effective ways to enforce the rules that limit treats and screen time; this part of being an enforcer can be a challenge.

Consistency is a key aspect of being an enforcer. If this means not following all of the 5 Simple Rules to perfection, that is okay. It is better to be consistent in whatever aspects we have chosen. When it comes to creating a healthy-weight home, doing a little all the time is more successful than doing a lot inconsistently.

Coach's Corner — Being a positive enforcer

Situation: Two of us coaches were talking about the concept of being an enforcer. Our concern was that the word "enforcer" can be taken negatively, sounding as if parents need to force children to eat a certain way. We wanted to make sure that we were able to help parents understand the importance of the role without going to extremes.

Strategies: In talking it through, we decided to describe the enforcer as a parent who makes the 5 Simple Rules come to life by turning potentially negative situations into positive ones.

This is best done by telling children what they can do, not what they are not allowed to do. For example, rather than telling a child not to drink juice at dinner, the enforcer might say, "Since you're thirsty, I'll get you some water." When offering snacks, the enforcer could ask the child to choose either an apple with peanut butter or some cottage cheese with fruit. Becoming this kind of enforcer tends to take lots of practice, so we decided to have the couples work together as a team to support each other's consistency in practicing the strategy.

Young children look to us as the source of food. They have a natural trust that they will be given the right foods in the right amounts and at the right times of the day. This trust shapes a child's attitudes about food. Kids are very self-involved and do not realize that their parents and caregivers have busy lives and need to make compromises as part of daily life. In one study, mothers reported having a hard time balancing the demands of family life with work, healthy eating, and maintaining a pleasant mealtime atmosphere at home. It is important to understand the trust our children put in us when it comes to food and to take that into account as we make food choices on a day-to-day basis. Focusing on consistently providing wholesome, nutritious foods for the whole family sends a powerful message to children at an early age.

As kids get older, the focus on consistency continues to be very important, and the types and amounts of food in the house affect the quality of everyone's diet. In one study, it was found that girls ate more fruits and vegetables simply because they were available at home. The same study found that easy access to less wholesome foods led to poorer food choices. Girls who had free access to soft drinks at home, for example, ate fewer dairy products.

(*Coach's Corner*)   **Enforcing treat rules**

Situation: Parents have a lot of questions about treats. Often I am asked what the best way is to enforce this rule.

Strategies: In my experience, these tried-and-true strategies are the most effective:

- Buy treat foods one serving at a time at a convenience store, gas station, or ice cream store, allowing children to pick out their treat for the day. One mother turned choosing treats into an afternoon activity by walking to the store and then having her children pick out something for themselves. She found that this approach kept her kids from fixating on treats when they were at home.

- Put treats in a closed container on a high shelf, not at eye level. There is a lot to be said for out of sight, out of mind.

- Encourage kids to choose their one or two treats for the day. They are much more careful when they can make their own decisions—for example, whether to have their cookie after school or before bed.

- Avoid pressuring children not to eat certain foods at friends' houses. Trying to enforce strict rules when the parent is not there usually backfires, with the kids eating more of the food than if it had never been mentioned.

Out of concern for our children, it is not uncommon for some of us to overdo the role of food enforcer. This rarely works. In fact, superstrict enforcement often backfires. Research finds that the eating habits of girls, in particular, are influenced in an unwanted way by parents (especially mothers) who are too strict about the foods they eat. At the end of the day, the enforcer role is all about balance.

In a healthy-weight home, everyone needs to follow the same rules and policies. While the 5 Simple Rules are simple, they are not easy. Many of us parents have trouble enforcing our own eating habits. We try to be too strict, too rigid, and too perfect in our eating habits, only to find that we have times of overeating as a consequence. These periods of overeating are called *dietary disinhibition*. Many of us are simply unaware of just how much our own patterns of food restriction and disinhibition affect the eating habits and weight of our children. One study finds that preschoolers whose mothers were disinhibited eaters had the hardest time with self-control around food. In another study, kids whose parents were on either end of the scale—being either highly restrained eaters or having a lot of episodes of disinhibited eating—had the most body fat as compared to preschoolers whose parents were neither. In addition, children whose parents said that they were both highly restrained and disinhibited eaters gained the most body fat during the preschool years.

How is it that our habits can have such a great effect on our children? In part, this is because as role models we teach kids both good and not-so-good eating behaviors. Often without realizing it, we may apply some of our own restrictive patterns to the way we feed our kids. This can cause children to lose touch with their body's hunger and fullness signals. To help children, it is useful to work on becoming more aware of our own food beliefs, attitudes, and habits. If being overweight is an issue, it may help to join an adult-based weight-loss program like Weight Watchers that emphasizes healthy eating practices, teaches positive thinking skills, and provides a supportive atmosphere. Having all the adults in the house follow the 5 Simple Rules also helps.

Coach's Corner   Money isn't everything

Situation: One of the women I work with was trying to create a healthy-weight home for her children only. She decided not to try to change her husband's eating habits since he comes home late from work and tends not to eat with the family. Usually, he picks up something to eat for dinner at the office. One night, she encouraged him not to eat before leaving the office and instead to eat at home. She had bought him fried chicken plus side dishes because she had a coupon. The children wanted to know why Dad was getting fried chicken and they were not.

Strategies: I explained that if she was serving fried chicken to her husband, she should expect that her children would want to eat it too. We discussed the importance of ignoring and getting rid of coupons for foods that do not fit a healthy-weight home, regardless of how much money they save.

Family meals are among the most important strategies to enforce as part of a healthy-weight home. Research shows that children who frequently eat family dinners are more likely to eat more fruits, vegetables, and dairy products. They are also more likely to eat breakfast.

A valuable enforcement strategy in a healthy-weight home is to turn off the television during mealtime. An increasing number of children watch television during meals and snacks, and this practice is linked with poor food choices. In one study, boys who watched television also asked more often for foods they saw advertised on television.

Family policies on a child's allowance can have a surprising effect on his or her eating habits. When children have a lot of their own money to spend, it can weaken their parents' efforts to limit treats. Grandparents, too, can be a source of spending money. Helping kids learn good money skills, as well as reinforcing the 5 Simple Rules by teaching kids how they can save for a highly valued item by not buying treats, is a strategy that works for many families.

As discussed earlier, calorie-containing beverages like fruit juice are a big source of excess calories for many kids. This is an area where enforcing a change can make a big difference by limiting these beverages to no more than half a cup per day. Not having soft drinks in the house and buying only small amounts of fruit juice is an effective strategy. Likewise, enforcing the practice that only low-fat or nonfat milk and water can be beverages for meals and snacks also works.

Infants

Because babies are completely dependent on us for food, enforcement at this age is automatic. However, many of us do not realize how much our own actions influence the eating habits and weight of an infant.

What works for infants is support from a spouse and other caregivers for the mother who decides to breast-feed her baby. Breast-feeding can become harder to keep up if the baby gets supplemental bottles of formula from other caregivers. The decision to breast-feed is a worthy one. Research finds that babies who are breast-fed drink fewer sweetened drinks and eat less added sugar as they get older.

Once an infant starts eating solid foods, baby foods without added salt, sugar, or fat are recommended. Enforcing this decision when others are feeding the baby is a good step to take.

What doesn't work is forcing the baby to feed for a set amount of time or to finish the bottle. Babies know their own appetite. They cry when they are hungry and lose interest in feeding when they are full. Helping infants keep their hunger and fullness cues intact is a great way to guide them toward eating the right amount of food in the years to come. Encouraging overeating makes babies unlearn these cues and want to finish everything.

Overly strict feeding does not work in older kids, and it does not work in babies either. While not buying baby foods with added sugars, salt, and fats is recommended, even infants can sense when restrictions are too tight. Certain foods become more appealing, especially if the child sees other family members eating them. Infants approaching their first birthday can begin to learn about treats and have them included as part of their daily life.

(*Coach's Corner*)   **Overrestriction backfires**

Situation: A father with two young children asked about how strictly he should enforce a no-sugar rule. His older child received no foods with sugar for the first year of her life. Her first taste of sweets was on her first birthday, when she tasted a cookie from the bakery that made her birthday cake. Two years later, she is a big lover of sweets. Dad wondered if he should be as strict with his second child since the strategy didn't work for his daughter.

Strategies: It could be that Dad was so strict about sugar with his daughter that she reacted by wanting and enjoying sweet foods more. We decided that he would try being less strict with his son. Enforcement would be harder anyway, because his son was exposed to treat foods during his sister's playgroup snack time. So far, it seems to be working, because his son does not have a sweet tooth and often does not finish his dessert.

Toddlers and Young Children

Many toddlers and young children can best be described as fussy. Saying no, refusing to eat, and otherwise defying adults is what they do best. Understanding that fussiness is part of a young child's normal development helps—as does coming up with new strategies and approaches to enforce healthy eating.

What works for toddlers and young children is enforcing food rules with gentle firmness. The effective enforcer tells the young child what the choices are, allows the child to pick, and does not react emotionally if the child says no or has a tantrum. As hard as it is to avoid reacting, a calm approach tells the child that you are in charge and that emotional outbursts will not change your mind.

Eating vegetables is a common battleground for young children.

Kids have a natural attraction to sweetness and they are sensitive to many of the strong flavors that are found in vegetables. It may take a lot of effort to raise a child who likes eating vegetables, but vegetables should be a consistent part of daily meals. By calmly including the same vegetable for several meals in a row without making a big deal about it, we can overcome the natural resistance many young kids have. Seeing the rest of the family eating vegetables also helps.

Coach's Corner   Kid pressure

Situation: A mother asked how she could limit the number of treat foods in the house without facing questions and nagging from her school-age children.

Strategies: One strategy that works for a lot of parents is not bringing children to the market during food shopping trips. Children spot foods they don't have at home and often pressure their parents to buy foods they prefer not to buy. Another strategy is to limit the shopping list to wholesome, nutritious foods that enforcers of a healthy-weight home want their children to eat. In this mother's case, when foods simply were not available in the home, spontaneous food fights were reduced dramatically.

Young children need snacks—their stomachs are too small to hold enough food in just three daily meals. An effective strategy is to think of snacks as minimeals for young children, providing the same foods that are given for breakfast, lunch, and dinner. Having this attitude, and enforcing it, helps children learn the difference between a snack and a treat.

Coach's Corner   **Snack/treat confusion**

Situation: I was told by a mother about her two young children who were confused. When they went to the houses of friends, they were given cookies or candy, and the food was called a snack. At home, a snack was fruit or a glass of milk. Mom asked for ideas on explaining the difference between snacks and treats to her children.

Strategies: We decided Mom should tell her children that the snacks at home are anytime foods that can be eaten whenever they are hungry. She explained that many of the foods that they are offered at friends' houses are really treats. While treats are okay, they are not anytime foods. When it was explained in this way, the kids got it.

Enforcing family meals that include the toddlers or young children in the house sets the foundation for family eating habits that will hold in the years to come. Family meals at this age also allow children to see how other family members eat. Research finds that children are more likely to eat fruits and vegetables if they see others eating them and if they are introduced by late infancy. The natural phenomenon of fear of new things that is common in young children is lessened when new foods are simply part of a family meal.

What doesn't work for toddlers and young children is absolute restrictions. At this age, limiting the use of soft drinks and fruit juices can be a particular challenge. Being overly strict can lead a child to prefer these foods and to drink them uncontrollably when they are available away from home. As a less rigid approach, some families have a policy that says that these foods are not served at home, but it is okay to have them when visiting friends.

> ### (Coach's Corner) Learning to manage soft drinks
>
> **Situation:** A father of three children asked me for help in enforcing a no-soft-drink rule at home for his three young children.
>
> **Strategies:** The first step for this father was to stop buying soft drinks for the house. Instead, he stocked up on low-fat milk and also encouraged his children to drink water. He explained to his children that he wanted the family to live in a healthy-weight home and that this was part of doing so. One day, his son came home from a friend's house feeling guilty because they had soft drinks. Dad explained that this was fine, that it was a treat and having treats is okay.

Experts strongly advise against putting young children on a diet to lose weight. Likewise, it is a good strategy not to make any comments about a young child's weight or body shape. In a group of young girls, those who had the highest levels of dietary restriction, were the most concerned about their weight, and were the most dissatisfied with their body had the greatest weight gain. In our role as food enforcer, we should look for alternatives to dieting—namely, focusing on the wholesome, nutritious foods that promote a healthy weight.

Older Children

Until they reach the rebellious teen years, older children are proof that enforcement of the 5 Simple Rules pays off. Most kids eat a variety of foods at this age and know the difference between wholesome foods and treats.

What works for older children, as with younger children, is consistent family meals. While schedules are always busy at this age, enforcing the policy of regular family meals is helpful. Studies find that older children are confident in their ability to choose wholesome foods. Family meals also provide the chance to applaud the wise choices that a child makes.

Coach's Corner   **Teens and family dinners**

Situation: A family's teenage daughter did not want to eat with the family. Her mom felt that including the daughter in family dinners would improve her eating habits and wondered if I had any suggestions for bringing teenagers back to the table.

Strategies: In talking with the mother, I found out that the daughter loved to cook. I suggested to Mom that she ask her daughter to pick out dishes that she would like to cook from cookbooks that focused on healthy recipes. The daughter had fun making the meals and took pride in eating them with her family. Mom used the family dinners to compliment her daughter's cooking skills and to help reinforce reasonable portion sizes for the entire family.

Family meals improve the health and well-being of older children far beyond their nutritional effects. One study found that children who ate meals frequently with their family were less likely to use tobacco, alcohol, and marijuana. The children in the study were also less likely to have a low grade point average or show symptoms of depression.

Coach's Corner   **Feeding hungry teens**

Situation: The mother of two teenage children wanted to be a strong enforcer. She focused on wholesome foods for the house and wanted to avoid fast-food meals for the family. Sometimes her children were so hungry after sports practice, though, that fast food was an attractive option.

Strategies: We talked about strict enforcement of a no-fast-food policy and I helped her to see that it was not a realistic goal for her family at this point in time. Instead, Mom and her children discussed fast-food choices ahead of time and thought about some wise food choices. Mom took care to stop short of telling her children what they could and could not order, because as soon as she said no, they would say yes. On the next trip to the fast-food restaurant, Mom was pleased when both children made the choices they had discussed. While this does not always happen, her kids are making those wise food choices more often than they ever did before.

What doesn't work is not making family meals a priority. Teens who eat meals frequently with their family think that family meals are important, and teens who eat family meals that take place in a pleasant environment are less likely to develop eating disorders. Researchers find that making family meals a priority, even when schedules are hectic, is the one thing that protects girls most against disordered eating and going on fad diets to lose weight.

Because consistency is such an important part of being a food enforcer, many find planning ahead makes the job easier. For example, keeping snacks and bottles of water in the car avoids unplanned stops at fast-food restaurants. Cooking and freezing foods on the weekend, preparing dinner foods early in the day with a slow-cooker, and using time savers like precut vegetables and meats make the goal of providing wholesome meals during the week doable.

Even more than younger kids, older kids benefit when family policies are enforced to keep weight-related comments off limits, including comments about a child's need to lose weight. Research finds that girls who restrain their eating or try extreme weight-loss methods are more likely to gain excess weight. Keeping the focus on living a healthy lifestyle and away from weight works best.

The Beal Family Story

by Cristina Beal

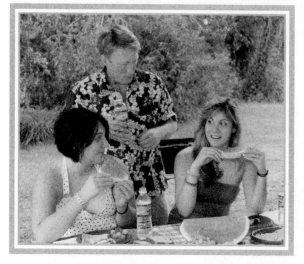

Cristina Beal's ex-husband and their two daughters having a healthy picnic lunch

Our family faces eating challenges a bit different from those of the typical two-parent family—I am divorced and my teenage girls spend time in both my household and the household of their father. We parents teamed up so that the girls' food environment stays consistent between the two homes.

In my role as an enforcer, my job is to make sure that the girls' father has access to the same information and guidance that I do. I make a copy of all the information I have regarding food—tips, recipes, game plans, and instructions—and give it to the girls' father. That way, he knows exactly what we are doing in my home and he can do the same in his.

At my house, I have made a lot of progress in focusing on wholesome, nutritious foods. By limiting what I buy to what is on my shopping list, we all eat healthier and do not snack on treats.

My food shopping is totally different now. I buy only what I want the girls and myself to be eating. I do most of my shopping in the outside aisles of the supermarket, where most of the foods—fruits, vegetables, meats, and dairy products—are fresh and not processed. I serve a lot of salads, green beans, and other vegetables, even though one of my daughters does not like vegetables. Hopefully, if I keep enforcing healthful eating her tastes will change. The girls' father has a far easier time stocking only healthy foods. He was always the healthier eater!

Another big change for us was in the area of fast food. We are on the go all the time and we used to stop for a fast-food meal on the way home to get something to hold the girls over. Now that we have made changes in the foods we eat at home, the girls are not as hungry between meals. We wait to eat until we get home and I cook a meal that is far better for us and more filling than fast food.

I don't monitor and enforce the girls' eating when they are away from home. When they are with their father, I know that they are eating about the same way that they eat at home. They have embraced the new way of eating and they really don't want to go back to their old habits.

Chapter 11

Sit Less, Move More

The last chapter gave the ins and outs of enforcing food rules, and that is certainly an important role in creating a healthy-weight home. But it's also helpful to keep in mind that only the first two of the 5 Simple Rules are about food. The next two rules deal with the calories-out side of the body weight equation. Activity enforcers play just as useful a role as food enforcers—if not more so—in making sure that everyone in the family is active. This chapter delves into the fine points of being an activity enforcer, including a profile of the Lisboa family.

What Is an Activity Enforcer?

As adults, when we think back to our childhood, many of us remember days filled with active fun. From riding bikes to sports leagues to running around the neighborhood with friends, there was always a lot going on.

Today's kids are not likely to be as active, because they have many more ways to fill their free time, many that do not require moving around. More than ever before, children need someone to remind, encourage, and enforce being active. "Go outside and play" was a phrase that many of us heard when we were growing up. In today's world, that phrase often sounds like "Turn off the television/computer/video game and go outside and play." Without encouragement, many kids would not be as active as they need to be. In taking on the role of activity enforcer, we play a very important role in creating a healthy-weight home for the entire family.

Good Activity Enforcers

- Manage the family's free time
- Limit screen time
- Encourage and support physical activity
- Create a parent-child relationship that includes activity

In creating a healthy-weight home, one way to enforce the 5 Simple Rules is to manage the family's free time. Being an authoritative parent means making sure that everyone limits screen time and includes activity in their day. Many of us, adults and children alike, need a push to get moving—that is part of the enforcer's role.

We effective enforcers of a healthy lifestyle let it be known that we are in charge of the family's activity. To do this well, we strike a balance between taking control and not being too strict or demanding. This can be easy to say but hard to do. One of the best strategies to make this happen is to link the roles of role model and enforcer. Telling kids what to do and doing it too gives parents authority and credibility. It helps a lot when children see their parents being active and limiting screen time, not just talking about it.

Just as with food, as parents we make all the difference as we lead our family members into changing their activity habits. One study compared two different ways to help kids change the behaviors that affected their weight. One group of children was taught directly by the researchers. For the other group, the parents were taught the new behaviors and they, in turn, taught their children. The children who were taught by their parents were more successful in making the changes. Not surprisingly, this group of kids also lost more weight.

Children do best when they have people to cheer them on and make them feel good about themselves. An activity enforcer can be a child's personal cheerleader who offers encouragement and support around being active. Beyond providing backup, embracing the idea that activity is an essential part of a healthy-weight home makes it a core family value. This is done by making and enforcing policies that ensure that activity is part of family life.

Physical activity can be enforced in several ways. One way is to discover the activities a child truly enjoys. Often the activities a parent enjoyed as a child—such as a father who played football or a mother who loved ballet—are not shared by children. It helps when these differences are respected. This can be done by putting aside our own preferences and being enthusiastic about whatever a child wants to do. It is clear that kids who enjoy their activities are more likely to stick with them. There are lots of options to choose from. Most communities offer a wide variety of activities for children or families, including classes, leagues, playgroups, and fun runs.

While encouraging kids to pick their activities, someone also has to be sure that their choices are doable and safe. That is another job of the activity enforcer. For example, while lifting weights is a fine activity for older children and adults, it is often not recommended for younger children. Seeking professional advice about evaluating what is appropriate is discussed in chapter 15.

The importance of picking the right activities cannot be underestimated. Children who have confidence in their abilities are more likely to include activity in their lives as they get older.

When a family is active together, it builds closeness. In one study, children were almost six times more likely to be active when both parents were active, as compared to children with two inactive parents. The researchers suggested that it was the combination of sharing activities with their parents and getting encouragement from their parents that motivated these kids to be more active.

Coach's Corner   **Encouraging participation**

Situation: A mother and father asked for suggestions for motivating their teenage son to be more active. Left on his own, the son did not seem interested in being active at all. He spent his free time in front of the computer.

Strategies: We came up with a long list of possible activities that the son might enjoy and have confidence in doing. The parents told their son they really felt he needed to be more active and then gave him their list of activities to choose from. Knowing that his choice was not *if* but *what*, their son decided to dust off his bike. He knew how to ride, but had not done it much since the computer had been put in his room. He started by riding short distances just to the corner and back. Then he started riding to the local park and back. There he met other teens in the neighborhood, who invited him to play basketball and football with them. Now, more afternoons than not, he is out of the house with his friends. After getting a lot of peer support, he even tried out for his school's basketball and football teams. He still loves his computer, but now uses it mainly for homework.

The flip side of encouraging activity is discouraging screen time. Television watching, video games, and computer time, collectively known as screen time, offer kids an appealing alternative to being active. That is why Rules #3 and #4 of the 5 Simple Rules work so beautifully together. Just as enforcers set and enforce the policies about activity, they are also the ones to create limits on screen time. One study found that over the course of their childhood, children with the greatest amount of television viewing gained the most body fat. Another concluded that being inactive, which included screen time, was directly related to excess weight in kids.

Medical organizations and professional groups all recommend that nonhomework screen time be limited to no more than two hours per day. And while this goal may seem unreasonable, it is based on the strength of the science that links screen time with excess weight in children. Looked at another way, the recommendation does not mean that limiting screen time to two hours has to happen overnight. Every small step at reducing the amount of time that kids spend in front of screens is a big accomplishment.

(Coach's Corner) **Cutting down on screen time**

Situation: A mother admitted that her son spent far too much leisure time in front of a screen. He played video and computer games at home and always brought his handheld video game with him on car rides and family trips. She asked for help in setting limits for her son's screen time.

Strategies: One of the 5 Simple Rules is to limit nonhomework screen time to less than two hours per day. Mom came up with the idea of letting her son bank screen time by spending less time playing video games during the week and saving the hours to use on weekends. She also began enforcing the need to be active every day. At first, her son kept track of his banked hours. But as time went on, he stopped being so concerned about how many minutes he had for the weekend. The mother was amazed at how far he had come when he started bringing a ball with him on family trips instead of his handheld video game.

The enforcer creates a healthy-weight home by motivating family members to be active. Studies find that children of parents who support their activity on all levels are more likely to want to be active and are confident about their physical skills. This is particularly true for more strenuous activities like jogging or jumping rope. Children are more willing to take part in higher-intensity activities when they believe in their physical ability to do so.

As parents, we are able to boost our children's self-efficacy—that is, their belief that they can do an activity—by making sure that they learn the physical skills that are needed, like how to hit a baseball, ride a bike, or swim. Research finds that a parent's involvement, including enthusiasm for the activity, instruction in the basic skills, and encouragement of the child's efforts, boosts self-efficacy. In boys, those with the highest levels of activity self-efficacy are the most active. Exercise and sports information from fathers has an extremely strong effect on the activity levels of their sons.

Decisions about how to spend family free time are a daily event. Creating household policies and practices that encourage activity is an effective strategy to get into the habit of moving. As with food, doing a little advance planning can make the job of activity enforcer a lot easier to accomplish. For example, having a game plan for what to do when the weather is bad can be very helpful, especially if most of the family's

(Coach's Corner)   **Adjusting to the change
in seasons**

Situation: The parents in an extremely active family were concerned about becoming inactive during the hot summer months. The family enjoyed many outdoor activities together—running, bicycling, in-line skating, and playing tennis. They asked me for some ideas that had worked for other families in the same situation.

Strategies: Using what others had told me to start the ball rolling, we quickly came up with several ideas that these parents thought might work for their family. The challenge was to get the school-age kids to agree. Mom and Dad first approached their children for more suggestions. Rather than pick new activities, the kids said that they would prefer to keep doing what they enjoyed but at a different time of the day. So, based on their kids' idea, Mom and Dad agreed to wake everyone up earlier in the morning for in-line skating or tennis.

activity is done outdoors. Having indoor activity options helps keep the family moving and away from screens. This is important because attending to both sides of the activity equation—increasing activity and reducing inactivity—is what research shows can help children lose body fat and increase their fitness levels.

One of the most effective strategies is to enforce family policies in ourselves. There is no question that parental inactivity affects the activity level of children. Inactive parents have a stronger effect on their child's activity than do parents who take part in vigorous physical activity—in other words, active parents do not guarantee active kids, but inactive parents are very unlikely to have active kids.

There is a strong connection between a child's overall activity level and how much time is spent outdoors. According to the Institute of Medicine, most children do not spend enough time outside. When outdoor time is enforced, children automatically get more active. Of course, it helps to have a place to play and equipment that promotes activity. Examples include swing sets and jungle gyms for younger children and a basketball hoop for older children. Local parks and trails are great places to be active as well.

Being more active is not just about playing games or being on a sports team. Having kids be more active through the use of chores is another effective strategy. Walking the dog, washing the car or windows, mowing the lawn, and raking leaves are all activities that can be assigned to a child. In deciding what chores to pick, it helps to choose them based on both their exercise value and the appeal they would have to the child who is being told to do them.

Community-sponsored sports are another option in the activity toolkit. One study found that when sports were made available in a community, the average number of girls and boys who participated in more vigorous physical activity increased. After-school programs, community centers, parks departments, religious institutions, and other community organizations offer activity options for children who live in the area.

Infants

Because infants cannot be active on their own, they need to have activity built into their days. This is particularly true in homes where the baby spends some or all daytime hours with a caregiver.

What works for infants is to provide caregivers, including sitters, daycare centers, and relatives, clear instructions about the activity expectations for a child. If there is to be little or no screen time while the child is with the caregiver, this needs to be stated. In addition, caregivers may need to be shown how to help the baby be active. As an infant gets older, caregivers can be taught new activities that the baby enjoys and be asked to include them in the daily routine.

What doesn't work is long periods of being in an infant seat, stroller, or crib, especially if it is in front of a screen. Activity helps babies develop the muscles and skills they need for sitting, standing, and walking. Infants who spend a lot of time being inactive miss out on the chance to build these vital skills. Inactivity sends a message at a very early age that movement does not need to be a part of each day.

Toddlers and Young Children

Toddlers and young children usually need to have boundaries set around being active and screen time. Creating a daily routine that includes lots of playtime and a little screen time gives young children a sense of familiarity and security. The job of activity enforcer tends to be easier when kids are young because they are more likely to go along with the rules, especially when the routines are consistent.

What works for toddlers and young children is to make sure that they get active, having playtime every day. Toddlers and young children are eager to play but need someone to plan the activity, find the space, and provide the toys. A strategy that works for many families is to set aside a specific time or times of day for play—in the morning after breakfast, after an afternoon nap, or before an evening bath. Likewise, having set times for television or videos at this age also helps.

Finding fun and practical play spaces can increase the amount of time a child will play. Helpful things to look for in local parks or playgrounds are toilet facilities, safety equipment, working water fountains, and shade. Areas that are close to home and offer organized activities for kids are an appealing option to many parents.

When the weather is bad, activity needs to move indoors. Favorite activities for young children include an indoor scavenger hunt or obstacle course. Both are easy to create and do not take a lot of time. If possible, a playroom or basement that can be equipped for hopscotch, hula-hooping, or a game of catch with a soft ball becomes a sought-after place by children on a rainy or snowy day.

Coach's Corner What to do in bad weather

Situation: A mother asked for ideas for activities on days when the weather is either too hot or too cold to take young children outside.

Strategies: Sometimes it takes creativity to come up with indoor activities that involve movement rather than screen time. This mother decided to create a CD that she and her children sang and danced to for thirty minutes on afternoons when outdoor play time was not an option. She felt better knowing that she had a fun and handy way to enforce activity no matter how bad the weather was.

It is clear that support encourages activity in young children. Support can be provided in many different ways. For example, young kids are likely to be active when they get logistical support, that is, being registered for activities, being supplied with balls and other play equipment, having play dates set, and being driven to lessons or classes.

What doesn't work is assuming that children will be active when they are under someone else's care. Preschools may not schedule in activity or may take the kids outside but not encourage active play. Caregivers in the home often require direction for including activity for a young child. One way to make sure kids are active is to arrange regular playdates and communicate that the kids should use them to play.

Televisions are becoming more common in the bedrooms of kids, and this practice is not helping the weight gain situation. In fact, preschool children who have a television in their bedroom are more likely to gain excess weight. Limits on television watching and screen time are much easier to enforce if the screens are limited in number and are kept in the home's living room or den. Having easy access to a television and total control of what is watched can actually encourage a child to be less active.

Coach's Corner   Activity does not offset screen time

Situation: Being a busy mother myself, I understood the situation described by one mother. Her young children participated in activities each day, so she felt that letting them watch television whenever they had free time was okay. She also used the television as a way to keep her kids entertained when she was too busy to spend time with them.

Strategies: The television may seem like an easy way to keep kids occupied, but I have found that many parents do not realize that the consequences of screen time include weight gain from a lack of activity. Unfortunately, some time spent in activity cannot be offset by a lot of time in front of screens. A healthy-weight household encourages both increased physical activity and decreased screen time. Knowing this, Mom understood why they are kept separate in the 5 Simple Rules and started to pay more attention to both factors.

Just as with food, promising a reward or treat for being active sends the wrong message to a child. This strategy may be effective in the short term, but eventually it teaches kids to see activity as a job that requires payment. The reward, which is often a food treat, becomes much more important and desirable.

Coach's Corner   **Walk for fast food**

Situation: One mother told me about her new strategy for getting her two young kids to be more active. They enjoyed eating fast food, so she promised them fast food if they would walk with her to the restaurant.

Strategies: I explained to Mom that children should not be bribed to be active. Kids do not need a reward to feel good about moving. A reward focuses their attention away from activity as something that is fun and enjoyable. Mom decided to come up with other fun destinations that the girls also enjoyed, like the local park, which did not have a link to food.

Older Children

Enforcing anything with an older child can be tough. Part of growing up is rejecting authority and challenging the decisions of adults. The trick for parents of older children is to find ways to motivate and encourage being active and limiting screen time without causing a rebellion.

What works with older children is providing welcomed types of support. For example, older kids often need help buying sports equipment. As parents, we can encourage activity by making sure that our kids have the right gear: a uniform that fits; shoes for the sport; a ball, glove, racquet, or other pieces of required equipment; and safety gear. Giving praise, showing interest, and attending events are also powerful tools that help motivate older children. By using these tools, parents show their teen that they have confidence in the teen's ability to do a particular activity.

Older children often form strong opinions about which activities they do and do not like. Supporting a child's choice of activities helps. Children who enjoy their selected activities, for example, a dance class for girls, are more likely to participate. In addition, children should be allowed to drop those activities that are no longer enjoyable and replace them with other ones—within reasonable limits, like once they have finished out the season.

Setting goals can help motivate older kids by giving them something concrete to work toward. Supportive strategies include talking about what is reasonable and achievable as well as helping to create a schedule with benchmarks to reach the goal. A child who reaches a goal feels rewarded and confident about striving for the next goal. This is one reason why the concept of achieving one's personal best is so strong in the area of activity.

While encouraging the use of goals for increasing activity, a similar strategy can be used with older children to reduce the amount of time spent being sedentary. Swapping sedentary time with active time works. One study showed that children who switched from sedentary activity to vigorous activity enjoyed being physically active more, and they also lost weight.

What doesn't work is being an enforcer without being a role model. Research shows that older kids are more likely to take part in after-school activities when both of their parents are active. In contrast, children whose parents watch more than two hours a day of television tend to be more sedentary. The enforcer's words do not work if they apply only to the kids and not to the adults in the home. The rules of limiting screen time and being active need to apply to all family members.

Older children are especially sensitive to criticism. Parents who make negative comments about their child's weight are more likely to have a child who dislikes sports and is less physical. Many families have a no-weight-comments policy in place, but it is up to the enforcer to ensure that the policy is carried out. This is time well spent.

Coach's Corner 5-2-1

Situation: One of the mothers in my group told me that she had shortened three of the 5 Simple Rules to the expression 5-2-1. The numbers stood for five daily servings of fruits and vegetables, no more than two hours of screen time, and at least one hour of physical activity. She ran into problems with the screen time rule because her husband had not agreed to cut down on watching television.

Strategies: Without her husband on board, cutting down on family television time was too difficult. Instead, she decided to focus on the activity side of the equation with the hope that it would overtake the inactivity side. She encouraged her husband to play soccer and walk around the school track with their children. She also planned active weekends and vacations filled with bicycle riding, family walks, and strolls along the beach. Often it is best to make the easier, doable changes first and tackle the harder ones gradually over time.

The Lisboa Family Story

by Myrna Lisboa

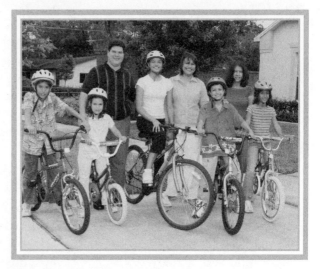

The Lisboa family loves to stay active

We have a lot of children in our household. My husband and I are raising three children: a teenager and two children in elementary school. My sister and her two elementary school–age children also live with us. All five children need to get daily physical activity. The three adults in the family need activity too! My sister and I are trying to control our weight, and my husband is overweight and has diabetes.

The kids in our family were not very active in the past and needed more exercise and physical activity. Once we learned about the importance of being active at least one hour a day, our daily routine really changed.

My sister and I make sure that the kids play outside at least one hour per day. The traffic on our street is dangerous, so the kids play in the backyard. They have a lot of different choices: jumping rope, kicking a soccer ball, playing baseball, and hula-hooping. I love to play with the kids when I can, but it is not always possible because I work. They know that they have to be outside every day, even if I am not home to remind them.

The kids also ride their bicycles from our house to a park that is two miles away. We had a truck that we used to drive the bikes to the park so that the kids could ride around. Once we sold the truck, the kids asked for permission to ride to the park and back. We said yes, and we join them when we can.

All of us have benefited from becoming more active. Our youngest child is a bit overweight. Since becoming more active, she has more energy and is happier. She used to be tired all the time, but not any more. My husband and I have both lost about 13 pounds. The other kids who do not have weight issues go to bed so much more easily because they are tired after the day's activities.

I know that I have not implemented everything I have learned. Every week, I've made little changes in the kids' routine and tried to do something new. I have found that small changes add up—the changes we have made have made a big difference in the kids' lives and in ours.

Chapter 12

Being on the Lookout

The roles of enforcer, provider, and role model take up the most time in creating a healthy-weight home. Two additional roles, however, also come into play. The first is that of being a protector. The second is to be an advocate. This chapter explores the role of protector and includes the story of Cara Geers, a woman who takes on the protector role both at home and in her job.

What Is a Healthy-Weight Protector?

One of the most important jobs we have as parents is to make sure that our children are safe, and many times this means taking on the role of protector. Protectors help keep children out of harm's way. This may mean standing up for a child if the child is being bullied; it may also mean fighting for a child's right to be treated fairly by teachers, coaches, and friends.

As parents, we create the family structure in which our children grow and develop. Children also learn about the social relationships that are part of community life through local events, churches, and neighbors. The relationships children develop within the community can be a strong support system as they grow older and have to deal with the trials and tribulations that come with life. Strong family structures and community relationships help keep our kids physically and emotionally healthy.

Good Healthy-Weight Protectors

- Guide how children deal with conflict
- Encourage activities and decisions that boost success
- Support children who have weight challenges

One of the first jobs of the protector is managing the relationships siblings develop with each other because these relationships affect the ability to sustain a healthy-weight home. It is not uncommon for children to deal with unresolved sibling conflict by rebelling against the 5 Simple Rules, and the protector has to make decisions about when and how much to get involved in kids' squabbles. Research suggests that parental intervention between young children is usually helpful and helps to keep the peace between siblings. Research also finds, though, that the relationship between older siblings actually tends to get worse when the parents get too involved.

In our role as protectors, we often take from our other roles—role model, provider, and enforcer—to be there for our own child or for other kids outside the home. Feeling protected by an adult is one way children learn how to navigate in the world in a safe and positive way.

Children are more likely to be successful when they are guided and encouraged to take part in family, school, and community activities. Parents help children make wise decisions for themselves. As a child grows older, parents need to gradually let go of the role of protector and let the child be more personally responsible for decisions and actions, including those related to the 5 Simple Rules.

While all children need protection, those with weight issues may have a greater need. It is sometimes hard to find the right level of protection to give a child. This is a tough issue, because giving either too much protection or not enough can create problems. It is known, however, that the most effective strategy is to treat all children in the family the same when creating a healthy-weight home. None of the children is helped by singling out a child who is overweight.

Coach's Corner — When one child is heavy

Situation: A mother and father were anxious to do something for their preteen who has weight issues. They asked for suggestions about how to work the 5 Simple Rules into the entire family's routine.

Strategies: I sensed that while the parents were committed to creating a healthy-weight home, they really saw it as a sacrifice that they had to impose on everyone for the sake of one child. I explained the reasons behind using healthy-weight strategies for the whole family and the benefits that everyone would get as a result. This helped them to see their efforts differently. As a result, they came to embrace the idea that weight, weight loss, body fat, and other weight-related words and subjects should be strictly off-limits at home. They knew that changing their lifelong patterns of treating their overweight child differently would be hard, so they decided to be on the lookout for each other when it came to overly enforcing the 5 Simple Rules with their heavy child and being more permissive with the other kids. In the end, they found that being consistent with everyone in the home made it easier to follow the 5 Simple Rules and cut down on weight-related bickering and name-calling.

One of the most challenging situations anyone can face is protecting a heavy child from the prejudice against excess weight. The sad reality is that children typically react less favorably to heavy children than to children of normal weight. In one study, children responded more negatively to drawings of heavy children today than they did in the early 1960s. This suggests that the stigma of excess weight in children is greater today than it was forty-plus years ago. The bias against excess weight can begin as early as preschool, with preschoolers preferring to play with a thin or average-weight child. Getting help from outside specialists who are able to assess the situation, including school guidance counselors and psychologists, can help. Chapter 15 provides information about getting professional help.

Coach's Corner   **Handling bullying**

Situation: The parents of a preteen boy told me that their son was being picked on and made fun of on the school bus because of his weight. As protectors, they wanted to find the best strategies for helping their son handle the situation.

Strategies: It really breaks my heart to hear stories like this and I could see how hurtful the bullying was, not only to the son but to the parents as well. After talking it through and getting insights from other parents who had had similar situations, the parents decided to try several different strategies. To learn more herself, Mom went to the library and read a variety of books on helping children handle bullying. She also found a youth support group for her son so that he would have peer support in handling the problem. Dad focused on spending more active time with his son—from bowling to hiking to doing yard work together—so that he could find out how his son was doing and also help him in his efforts to manage his weight.

Coach's Corner   **Diabetes in the family**

Situation: A mother approached me about changing her family's habits. Diabetes runs on her husband's side of the family (Dad has type 2 diabetes), and she was especially concerned about one daughter who was built just like her dad. While Mom's concern was for this one child, she did not want to single her out.

Strategies: I congratulated Mom on her commitment to adopting a different lifestyle for the entire family, not just for one child. While her heavy daughter may be more at risk for developing diabetes, by taking action now she was helping the other children as well. After some discussion, Mom decided never to mention weight as a reason for shopping and cooking differently—buying 100% whole wheat bread instead of white and putting more fruits and vegetables on the menu. Instead, she told the family that she simply wanted all of them to be healthier and was taking special care for Dad. Her strategy worked. Her daughter lost weight without trying and talks about having more energy during the day. In addition, all the kids are learning the importance of eating wholesome foods and being active every day.

Another way to protect our children, especially young children, is to shield them from situations that work against the 5 Simple Rules. Often these situations are related to specific people—for example, a grandparent who thinks that treats are a good reward or a friend who openly makes comments about a child's weight. Situations can also arise from a hectic schedule, like erratic days that are overfilled with activities so that meal and snack times are missed. A protector steps in on behalf of a child to minimize how often these situations occur and works to find new strategies that will help the child live by the 5 Simple Rules.

(*Coach's Corner*)   **Defending healthy eating**

Situation: A father was not sure how to help his teenage son. The family had committed to following the 5 Simple Rules and his son was making a lot of progress, but now the son's friends were making fun of him for eating healthy foods when they were eating lunch at school or hanging out in the evening. They tried to tempt him to eat what they were eating and be one of the gang. When the son went to his Dad for advice, the father was unsure what to tell him.

Strategies: We discussed the best strategies for protection against outside influences like unhelpful friends. Because the boy was older, we decided that a frank father-son talk about the situation made the most sense. In talking with his son, Dad discovered that his son was proud that his eating habits were giving him a healthier body and he wanted to continue. Dad encouraged this thinking and coached his son to keep his long-range goal in mind when he was spending time with his friends. Dad also reminded his son that just because his friends were thinner than he was did not mean that they were healthy. With his confidence and commitment bolstered, the son was able to better deal with his friends' comments.

In creating a healthy-weight home, taking on the role of protector helps to boost and maintain the self-esteem of a child with weight issues. It is not uncommon for kids with excess weight to have a lower self-image and sense of self-worth when compared to kids at a healthy body weight. Regardless of weight, self-esteem tends to get lower as children enter their teen years. This is important because poor self-esteem is linked to greater feelings of sadness, loneliness, and nervousness, along with a greater likelihood of smoking and drinking alcohol. Children with a low self-worth can also develop behavior problems. This can become a vicious cycle, because a child's negative feelings can dampen the motivation to follow the 5 Simple Rules. An effective strategy in these situations is to be sure to recognize a child's efforts and progress in following the 5 Simple Rules as a way to bolster self-esteem.

In our role as protector, we can have a big impact on the level of physical activity a child develops over time. Research shows that an active childhood often leads to continued regular physical activity through the teen years and into adulthood. Lifelong physical activity brings with it both weight and health benefits, including a lift in emotional well-being.

Protectors help find activities that are both age- and weight-appropriate for children. Physically, very overweight children are different from kids at a healthy weight and often have a limited ability to exercise. Because their bodies are larger, they have to work harder than a thinner child to do the same activity, and this leads to feelings of fatigue in a shorter amount of time. Heavier children are also more likely to have lasting effects from sprains and other activity-related injuries. While encouraging activity is certainly a part of having a healthy-weight home, pushing a heavy child to perform at a greater level in an effort to speed weight loss is likely to backfire and may, in fact, cause injury.

Activity is not just about physical ability, though—it is also a social event. Girls in particular say that body size and fear of negative comments from peers can keep them from being active. They may be embarrassed to exercise around their friends or refuse to wear shorts or a swimsuit. In these situations, encouraging activities that do not need a special outfit and can be done alone, like walking, biking, or using an exercise videotape, often works.

(**Coach's Corner**)   **Finding the right fit**

Situation: A mother and father told me how frustrated they were with the fitness options in their community. Their preteen, who was very self-conscious about his weight, was highly motivated to become more physically active but did not feel that he had any options open to him. The fitness program at the community's recreation center was filled with children who were much younger than he was. He was too young to use most of the exercise equipment at his local Y. And he was not interested in playing on a team until he got into better physical shape.

Strategies: It was clear that this child wanted to be active but was running into roadblocks in trying to make his goal a reality. In talking with his parents, we discussed how one effective way parents can protect their children is by speaking up. This couple decided to approach the Y and community center about starting a program for preteens with weight issues. They also explored the possibility of hiring a personal trainer to help their son get started with an activity routine. They planned to explore family activities like bicycling and walking. With several choices available to him, the son felt that the goal of being active in a way that suited him was possible.

What works is helping a child to boost self-esteem in the most sensitive areas. In one study, children with weight issues had lower scores relating to self-worth, physical appearance, and acceptance by their peers, but average scores for academic ability, athletic ability, and behavior. Focusing on a child's strengths and building up areas of weakness by providing a healthy-weight home makes a difference, as does cheering the child's efforts to get to a healthy weight.

Expressing confidence in a child's physical abilities also works. Research shows that the child of a confident parent feels that the parent is supporting his or her activity and the child becomes more motivated to continue. Moreover, when children are confident of their physical abilities, they are more likely to participate in activities. It also helps if the child finds the activities to be fun, a factor that is closely linked with a child's desire to participate.

Coach's Corner   **Fun without competition**

Situation: A mother and father of two children admitted to me that they were stumped. They never had to look for activity for their son because he was a competitive athlete who played on several teams. The challenge was their daughter, who did not enjoy sports competition. Mom and Dad were not sure where to turn for alternative activities for their daughter. The only activity programs that they knew about were teams through the town recreation department.

Strategies: Sometimes all it takes is a couple of phone calls to gather information. Mom and Dad made a few calls and talked to people about nonteam activity options. They found a noncompetitive soccer league that their daughter joined and enjoyed because it was low-key and relaxed. She felt successful playing on a team without the pressure of winning. She also took up horseback riding, an activity she now loves.

Being a protector means finding and encouraging realistic activity options. One way to do this is to organize family activities rather than persuade a child to join a group of peers. Family activities can build up the child's endurance and confidence while promoting family togetherness. The role of support cannot be underestimated. In a study of girls with weight issues, many said that limited adult support was a barrier to their being active.

Helping kids feel less insecure about their appearance is a form of protection. In one study, girls said that one of the main reasons they were not physically active was that they were self-conscious about their appearance. Community activity resources, including group classes geared toward heavy children, lessen this concern because everyone in the group has the same issue so nobody needs to be apprehensive about how he or she looks.

It helps to explore all the activity options that are available in a community. The school district, community center, Y, or school psychologist may offer a support group to help children handle the social aspects of excess weight. Support groups may lessen a child's concerns and boost self-esteem.

Coach's Corner — Cupboard makeover

Situation: A mother and father wanted to revamp the foods in their kitchen to make it easier for them to lose weight and to help one of their children, who was heavy. Their other two children did not have weight issues.

Strategies: We discussed the importance of creating a healthy-weight home for all members of the family, not just for the family members with weight concerns. Dad agreed to stop bringing in favorite foods that were low in nutrition and high in calories. Mom changed her attitude toward beverages, switching to water and calorie-free beverages and away from soft drinks. The refrigerator got stocked with healthy snacks like baby carrots, hard-cooked eggs, fat-free puddings, and fruit cups. Everybody in the family ate the same foods.

What doesn't work is trying to improve a child's social acceptance by explaining that the child has a medical problem. Research finds that while younger children may be more accepting of a heavy child with health issues, older children tend to react in a negative way.

It is also important to respect a child's experience with peers. Several studies find that many overweight children feel excluded from social circles and have fewer friends. While meant to be helpful, comments like "Everybody likes you because you have a great personality" do not change a child's social situation or improve his or her feelings of isolation. It is better to listen with empathy and support for the child's feelings rather than make comments that will not alter his or her experience.

Bullying is a real threat that should not be ignored. Overweight children are often the victims of bullying behaviors like rumor spreading, name-calling, teasing, or physical contact. All adults can and should protect a child against bullying. Strategies that have worked for parents of bullied children include reading books on the topic, joining a support group, and seeking professional help to help the child overcome weight-related bullying.

Knowingly or unknowingly, extended family members and friends can sabotage a family's efforts to create a healthy-weight home. While parents enforce the 5 Simple Rules within the family, they may also need to shield the family from others who are not supportive of the concepts. In addition, protectors have a responsibility to clearly communicate the house rules to caregivers, extended family members, and other frequent visitors. One area that often needs explaining with extended family members is a house policy against using food treats as a reward or gift.

(Coach's Corner)　**The well-meaning father**

Situation: A mother told me how frustrated she was with her ex-husband. He was so thrilled that his daughter wanted to go to the market with him that he agreed to buy her any food she wanted. When she asked him for a packaged pasta dish that was not particularly wholesome or nutritious, he bought several packages.

Strategies: I reminded Mom that, as a protector, it was her job to make sure that her ex-husband understood her desire to maintain a healthy-weight home. To do this, she explained to her ex-husband that focusing on wholesome, nutritious foods was a priority at home. If the pasta dish was going to be a treat for the day, that was okay. However, buying several packages gave the message to the daughter that this was an anytime food. He understood and said that he would make more of an effort to support the practice in future shopping trips.

Whether or not they require gym classes, schools are not a reliable source for physical activity. Even when physical education is available, children with weight issues may avoid joining in because of concerns about their appearance. Time needs to be set aside outside of school hours to ensure that activity takes place.

Coach's Corner   **Limited activity options**

Situation: The parents of a teenage girl were frustrated by her lack of activity. She had played soccer for several years but had become too old for the league. She enjoyed the local Y for a short period of time, then lost interest, and physical education classes were not offered in her school. After-school activity was difficult to schedule because school ends so late. Her parents were extremely active and wanted her to join them. They were not sure where to begin.

Strategies: Often, teenagers are not interested in doing anything with their parents, including activity. I suggested that Mom check with the high school and community recreation department about evening or weekend activities specifically for teens. Some teens enjoy taking walks as a way to get out of the house and spend time alone. The parents sat down with their daughter and told her that being inactive was not an option and then presented her with a list of choices that appealed to her. Though not overjoyed, she increased her activity level by taking a walk after dinner each evening.

The Geers Family Story

by Cara Geers

Cara Geers and her son

As the recreation superintendent of a parks and recreation department, I am in the fitness business. That is why it is so important for me to be the protector for my family, as well as for kids in the community.

My role as protector is to teach my son lifelong habits so that he does not face the same weight issues I did. I was husky throughout my childhood, and because I was extremely athletic, my mother let me eat everything. She did not realize that being active alone would not automatically make me a healthy weight. Once I did not have the time to be as active, I gained a lot of weight because I never learned how important it was to eat wholesome, nutritious foods and get physical activity every day. I had to protect my son.

I am a big supporter of my son's participation in sports. He has become confident and self-assured about his abilities in part because he knows that his parents are behind him all the way. I also focus on having wholesome, nutritious foods in the house as a way to protect him from developing an unhealthy diet. Despite my own experience, it was an eye-opener for me to realize that just because my son was fit did not mean that he could eat whatever he wanted. Thin does not equal healthy, and extra ice cream is not a reward for being thin.

I enjoy being able to use my skills as a protector with the children and parents I meet through my work. My favorite advice to parents is that children have to be involved with something outside of school. If they are not into sports, they should pick another activity, like scouts, music, or a cooking class for kids. Parents need to protect their children from an inactive lifestyle and from spending free time being sedentary.

One day I made a list of things that families could do in our community as part of a healthy, active lifestyle. The number of options was mind-boggling. Activities for parents included coaching a sports team, participating in a fund-raising walk, chaperoning a school dance, joining an adult sports league, starting a garden, joining the school PTA to help protect the eating habits and physical activity of kids, and volunteering to bring healthy foods to class parties. Families could participate in a fun run, do a family walk, take a parent-child karate class, and enjoy the city pools with discounted pool passes. We even offer a noncompetitive swim team for children who prefer more relaxed organized sports.

My husband and I are very active in team sports and in activities that we do individually, together, and as a family. I know that being a protector as well as a role model will help my son and the children in our community to grow up healthier.

Chapter 13

Taking It outside the Home

An advocate is someone who takes commitment to an issue to the next level. Taking on the role of advocate goes beyond what a protector does by actively seeking change. Advocates bring the principles of a healthy-weight home beyond the home and into the community. This chapter explores the many ways that an advocate can make a difference and introduces you to two of Dr. Lane France's colleagues who, as physicians, take their roles as advocates very seriously.

What Is a Healthy-Weight Advocate?

Today's kids live in a complicated world, with many factors that affect their health and well-being. The influence of a lot of those factors extends beyond the four walls of home. Kids do not have much say in how the world treats them, so they rely on adults to act on their behalf.

One important way that we as parents can be advocates for a healthy-weight home is to network with other parents to see what they are doing. Going further, there is the possibility of being an advocate within the community—supporting activities in the local parks and recreation department and volunteering for school events that are linked with food and exercise. Parents are not the only people who can be healthy-weight advocates, however. The role of advocate can be taken on by other family members, teachers, organizations in the community, and doctors.

As with any issue, healthy-weight advocates are most successful when we band together and work toward common goals. We can look at other public health issues to see what has worked and what programs have made a difference in changing people's behaviors. Just a few examples include the campaigns to reduce smoking, to increase the use of seat belts, and to have a designated driver. Each of these public health issues has had strong advocates working together to make a difference. Those advocates have made a lot of progress over the years, and the lessons that they have learned can be a valuable road map for those of us working to encourage achieving a healthy weight.

The changes that are most likely to reverse the trend in childhood obesity need to take place in two different arenas. The first is the environments in which we live on a day-to-day basis, including our homes, schools, and communities. The second involves the larger world, with big-picture issues like the food supply, food marketing campaigns, and national education standards. Advocates tend to be most effective when they focus on a specific issue and work at the level with which they are most comfortable.

Ways to Be an Advocate

We parents are the natural health advocates for our children. Most children do not have the age, maturity, knowledge, or earned respect to be their own advocates. Some of the most common examples of healthy-weight advocacy occur in the local schools. As the result of feedback and pressure, many school districts are taking another look at their decisions to not require physical education classes or to sell soft drinks in the cafeteria. One easy way to be an advocate is simply to vote for school board candidates who share your beliefs on these policies and practices. For those who want to be more involved, options include attending and speaking up in school board meetings, setting up discussion groups with other parents and school administrators, and joining committees. Importantly, being a healthy-weight advocate outside the home shows a commitment to the issue as it affects all family members.

What works is to join together with others to celebrate each small step family members make toward achieving a healthy weight. One group of researchers conducted a series of studies to see the impact adults had on the activity levels of children in the community. They discovered that children were more likely to participate in school fitness activities if both their parents and teachers encouraged them. In turn, the teachers believed that having parents who were committed to the fundamentals of a healthy-weight home was essential. Teachers were more likely to join parents on behalf of advocating for their children if they knew that there was commitment at home. In other words, healthy-weight practices at home can strengthen the parent-teacher team to the benefit of the child.

Besides working with teachers, asking other adults to support a child is a form of advocacy. Children's lives are influenced by many adults, including coaches, scout leaders, religious leaders, and others who are in a position to help.

Coach's Corner   **Coaching the coach**

Situation: One of the fathers I met was a coach for a recreation department sports team. He realized that he had an influence not just on his son, but on the other players on the team as well. He asked for tools, suggestions, and support to help him succeed.

Strategies: The first step I encouraged Dad to take was to increase his own understanding of the 5 Simple Rules. While he was fully supporting his wife's efforts at home, he had not taken the time to know the specifics. He quickly found that these were simple messages that he could share with his team. For example, he began pointing out how their practices were helping the kids get the hour a day of activity that their bodies need. He also recognized that as an advocate, he had the opportunity to pass on the same messages to the other coaches as well as to the parents of players on his team.

What doesn't work is when words and deeds are inconsistent. For example, advocating for healthier foods in the school cafeteria but then sending treats for a school event undermines the effectiveness of advocates. Classroom events that include supplying a snack can be the perfect opportunity to show commitment by sending in wholesome foods, like air-popped popcorn, homemade trail mix, yogurt parfaits, or vegetables with a low-fat dip.

Coach's Corner   Changing school foods

Situation: One mother was interested in working to change the way that lunch was handled at her children's school. The school did not have a cafeteria or space for preparing food. Each day, the staff brought in lunch from area fast-food outlets. The week's offerings—pizza, burgers and fries, fried chicken, and chicken nuggets—were not consistent with the wholesome foods that Mom was serving at home.

Strategies: Offering to be part of the solution is a great way to be an effective advocate. This mother volunteered to work with the school's food committee to explore ways to bring more wholesome foods in for school lunch. She started by suggesting small steps, for example, switching from regular chips to baked chips and serving ice cream just once a week instead of every day. She looked at the menus from the area fast-food chains that provided food to the school and highlighted better options, like yogurt-fruit parfaits, individual packages of fruit slices, and salads with low-fat dressing. Mom also identified additional quick-serve restaurants in the area that offered foods like sandwiches and roast chicken. The school expanded its lunch offerings to include these restaurants. Since the changes have been made, Mom has noticed that her children and their classmates are eating more wholesome meals in school as a result of her efforts.

Schools as Advocates

Enlisting educators to be healthy-weight advocates makes sense. Children spend as many waking hours in school as they do at home. As parents, we expect schools to take care of our children, looking out for their health and well-being as well as their academic education.

What works is to encourage good communication between the school and home. Through parent-teacher conferences, newsletters, or a note from the teacher asking to discuss a health-related issue at home, schools have many opportunities to keep the lines of communication open between the classroom and home. One study found that a combination of school and home improvements in health behaviors led to lower gain in body fat for both healthy-weight and overweight students.

Asking for changes in the food choices kids make at school can help them eat fewer calories overall. Wholesome, nutritious foods are both filling and lower in calories. Lower-calorie versions of popular foods—baked chips, lower-fat frozen desserts, and reduced-fat cheeses—supply fewer calories without compromising flavor. Schools are in the position to provide these foods to their students.

It is important to recognize the efforts all schools make to provide a solid education and develop their students' ability to learn. A child's weight and eating habits may affect learning success. One study found that overweight young adults were more likely to have learning problems, have grades that were below the class average, and/or require special education services than their healthy-weight classmates. Because weight loss enhances self-esteem and confidence, it may also have a positive effect on academic performance—a fact that schools may want to consider.

What doesn't work is to encourage schools to be overly zealous in imposing changes in their food service. Just as at home, small steps are more likely to lead to long-lasting change. Schools are more likely to be successful if they let students get used to small changes over time. Dramatic change can have students rebelling against being forced to choose wholesome, nutritious foods.

(*Coach's Corner*)   **The cafeteria slims down**

Situation: As a coach who encourages parents to advocate for wholesome foods in their children's schools, I was pleased to hear about a group of parents who had pushed their children's school cafeteria to replace most of their foods with healthier alternatives, like brown rice instead of white rice, sugar-free yogurts, light frozen desserts, and vegetarian entrées. After such radical change, however, the students complained that they had "nothing to eat" at school and either skipped lunch or brought snacks from home. The food service department began losing money and abandoned the changes.

Strategies: Looking back, a better approach would have been to make smaller changes over time and to wait a bit between each change to allow students to adjust. A coordinated effort involving the district's food service department, teachers, parents, and students might have led to a more favorable outcome.

Schools that place a very high value on team sports and activities that require a high skill level risk losing those students who do not want to or cannot participate. This is unfortunate, because school is an obvious place where children can be physically active if they are given the time and opportunity. Advocating for recreational teams within the schools and working to find sources of community support to fund the teams can reduce this risk.

Physicians and Health Care Providers as Advocates

Asking physicians and other medical professionals to become healthy-weight advocates can make a difference in the lives of many families. The frequent visits during the first few years of a child's life offer an opportunity to establish a solid relationship with a child's physician. As children get older, physicians and health care providers can spot potential health and weight problems and direct families to programs and services that will help them create a healthy-weight home.

What works is to get health care providers to make weight a routine part of visits and annual checkups. Quick office procedures like taking a child's height and weight, calculating BMI, tracking the BMI-for-age on a growth chart, and measuring a child's arm skinfold to evaluate body fat can be included in routine care. Providing feedback on the results helps. As a healthy-weight advocate for your child, it is reasonable for you to ask that these procedures be done and the results shared.

Health care professionals are respected for their expertise. Asking them to share the 5 Simple Rules with their patients helps spread the word.

What doesn't work is when a physician approaches weight-related behaviors in a critical way. Neither does it help when health care professionals avoid talking about their concerns with a child's weight or rate of weight gain because they are afraid of hurting the child's feelings, angering the parents, or sparking an eating disorder. Pediatricians are more likely to become healthy-weight advocates if they are asked for information and advice. One simple step is to ask about a child's BMI-for-age and how it has changed since the last visit. Taking this step demonstrates a commitment to the child and invites help from the child's doctor.

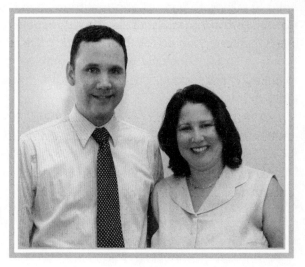

The Pediatric Healthcare Alliance Physicians

by Dr. Rick Wilde and Dr. Jackie Hartman

We are very concerned about excess weight gain in today's children. Millions of children in the United States weigh too much. In our opinion, excess weight gain is the number-one health threat to kids. Socially, children who weigh too much face discrimination, stereotyping, and poor self-esteem—all as a result of their weight.

We follow the weight guidelines of the American Academy of Pediatrics when working with patients. We plot BMI for every child in the office; this is as important as height and weight. Our goal is to raise awareness among parents that weight management is important.

A family-based approach to healthy weight is essential because weight issues, treatment, and prevention affect the entire family. We work together with parents to teach them how to create a healthy lifestyle for their family. Parents buy the food and create the eating environment, so they have to be in control of nutrition for the family. The first place to start is with the parents' own habits. Parents can't tell children to eat more healthfully and then sit down with a bag of chips. Parents have to be role models for their children.

Nutrition guidance is a part of every appointment because children need to develop good habits from the start. In the office, we make a point of talking to parents about nutrition and healthy eating for their kids, but not about weight loss. We recommend preventive strategies like not offering solids for the first four to six months, limiting juice, avoiding soda, choosing water and milk as preferred beverages, selecting snack food wisely, eating regular meals, avoiding fad diets, and keeping active.

Advice is the same for all parents, regardless of their child's BMI. Parents of healthy-weight children are often surprised that good nutrition is just as important for their healthy-weight children as for heavy children.

We convince busy parents that they always should make time for important family issues like healthy weight. Now is the time to advocate for children—their weight issues are not their fault and they cannot advocate for themselves.

Parents can be a valuable resource. We believe that parents are natural role models for kids; if parents live and create a healthy lifestyle, children will do the same as they grow up. Children really do want to please their parents. By serving as role models, parents show them how.

As advocates, we encourage parents to advocate for their children in the schools. Parents have to let school districts know if they are against low-nutrition foods and soft drinks in the cafeteria. Parents need to discuss with school districts the importance of putting physical activity back into the daily schedule. Wholesome foods, limited screen time, and physical activity at home are even more important when schools fall short.

We wish we had known how to eat when we were children. It would be great if we all learned about a healthy lifestyle during childhood. Good eating and activity habits are learned behaviors that last a lifetime.

PART THREE

Special Circumstances

While every family has the power to work toward a healthy-weight home, it is easier for some than for others. Many families have circumstances that make the job more challenging. The final section of this book addresses some of those issues—from having an unsupportive partner to parenting a child with disabilities.

Weight Watchers is not a medical organization; its weight-loss programs and services are based on good science and recommendations that are geared for the general public. The 5 Simple Rules and the five roles that parents play were developed with this in mind. Everyone's circumstances are different and none of the information provided in this book can or should replace guidance from the health care professionals who work directly with your family.

Fortunately, there are many professional resources available to help families working toward living a healthy lifestyle. The last chapter provides information about available professional resources—what they are, what they do, and how to find them.

Chapter 14

Few Families Are Traditional

Creating a healthy-weight home is within the reach of every family, but some families have more challenges than others. This chapter explores some special situations and provides insights into the impact they have on following the 5 Simple Rules.

Many families do not fit the definition of a traditional family. Many families have at least one child with a physical, health, or mental disability. Other families have living arrangements where the kids live with one parent. Or the kids may live part time with both parents in separate households (often as part of a blended family). Other kids live with one parent as a miniunit within an extended household that includes grandparents, aunts or uncles, and an employed caregiver like a sitter. In today's world, there are many, many definitions of a family home.

Regardless of the definition, every home can be a healthy-weight home. This can be done by following the 5 Simple Rules and having the adults who live in the home be positive role models, providers, enforcers, protectors, and advocates.

Children with Disabilities

The extra help that children with disabilities need to reach a healthy weight is both specialized and broad. Regardless of the type of disability (i.e., learning or physical), experts stress that the weight-related goals for children with disabilities need to go along with the larger goals for the child, including:

- Promotion of normal growth
- Maximal opportunities to develop to the child's potential
- Learning positive eating habits that will last into adulthood
- Encouragement to be active
- Development of social skills with family members and those in the community

In other words, while having a healthy (or healthier) body weight is a worthy goal for a child with special needs, it needs to be balanced with other child-centered goals too. Getting the advice of experienced health care professionals (discussed in chapter 15) can be a good strategy to help decide just how important a child's excess weight is in relation to other issues he or she may face.

Closeness within the Family Is Key

All children are affected by the contacts they have with others inside and outside their homes. The sensitivity of these relationships is naturally increased when a child has special needs.

Research shows that it is not uncommon for a parent to be upset if she thinks her special-needs child is being singled out or is not being respected by others. It is also common for the parents of a disabled child to feel isolated.

The source of these feelings is well founded. The activities of a special-needs child often require advance planning and this fact may be seen by others as a hassle. This is particularly true as a child gets older and social plans are made by the peer group. The social lives of children tend to be spur-of-the-moment, and because of the need to plan ahead for a special-needs child, peers may exclude the child from last-minute outings. The lack of an invitation can play into the feelings of isolation.

It helps to understand what is happening and give empathy, support, and encouragement. One way to do this is to pay special attention to having family meals. Research shows that regular family meals that include the involvement of the special-needs child can boost family closeness and help reduce parents' stress levels.

Parents often ask . . .

Is there anything I can do to lessen my child's feelings of isolation?

With your child's permission, it may help to plan activities and then invite others to join your child rather than waiting for invitations to come in. By doing this, you accept the responsibility for the planning, removing it as a barrier to your child's being part of a social gathering.

There are other ways to boost family closeness as well. Studies suggest that having both parents involved in a child's therapy enhances the parental relationship and helps a child's progress. In addition, parents who have a child with special needs report that despite the increase in stress that having a special-needs child brings, they have an increased feeling of family closeness and are more sensitive to the differences in others. This experience helps them to be especially effective advocates.

Families don't just include adults. Siblings who know about and understand their brother's or sister's disability have an improved attitude, better mood, higher self-esteem, and stronger feelings of social support. A sibling's knowledge about the special-needs child also works to create higher levels of family closeness.

Nontraditional Family Structures

Divorce is the biggest reason for nontraditional families. According to government statistics, 85% of children lived in a two-parent home in 1970. By 2000, the percentage dropped to 69%, with more than one quarter (26%) of all children living with one parent, usually their mother.

Lifestyle Changes

Splitting up households affects several aspects of a child's food and activity routines. Being a single head of a household often means that money is tight, and tighter finances affect the ability to be a provider. The amount of money that can be spent on groceries may be limited, as is the ability to pay for participation in activities like dance classes or a club sport.

Establishing a new household, however, often brings the opportunity to create a fresh start, including adopting the 5 Simple Rules. A new living arrangement provides the opening to buy different foods, set new meal times, and change family policies around screen time and activity. Moving to a new neighborhood gives the family a reason to shop at new markets, explore local parks, and try new restaurants. Parents can enforce new rules and be a food and activity role model. They may also be able to spend more free time with the kids.

A new home, whether the result of divorce, the death of a parent, or other reasons, has an impact on the psychological well-being of a child. Separation from one parent can reduce the contact with that parent's extended family. If that contact was positive and supportive, the child may feel abandoned. The child may not talk about the stresses that come with going from a two-parent household to a one-parent household; he or she may keep it inside. When this happens, it is not uncommon to see a negative change in attitudes around food and activity. These types of changes are cause for concern because kids who develop a negative opinion of themselves are at greater risk of developing disordered eating habits. Getting advice and guidance from an outside expert in these situations is always a good idea. Chapter 15 provides information on what to look for when seeking professional assistance.

Single Parenting

Many single parents face unique challenges when it comes to creating a healthy-weight home. Besides limited funds, they may have less time to focus on the five roles that are such an important part of living by the 5 Simple Rules. A lack of time can make it harder to provide wholesome, nutritious meals and snacks. Regardless, making as much time as possible to create a healthy-weight home is worth it and may improve a child's health.

Family togetherness also makes a big difference. A survey of mothers and their children aged ten to fourteen found that family closeness was the best predictor of having positive health habits. Other factors linked with health included family pride, general self-efficacy (having the confidence to take action and believing that success is possible), self-control, and a support network.

Parents often ask . . .

My life just does not allow me to eat dinner every night with the kids. Does that make me a bad parent?

Not at all. Family meals do not have to be dinner and they do not have to happen every day of the week. If dinner does not work, then try breakfast. Even having breakfast together on Saturday mornings or dinner together on Sunday nights can make a difference. If you have several kids in the house and getting them together is an issue, sitting down to eat with them individually is also an option.

Enforcing a commitment to family meals is a great strategy to promote family togetherness. Families who continue to eat meals together improve their chances of good health. Mealtime is the best time to be a food role model. Eating meals together may also enhance the health and well-being of adolescents. In one study, teens who ate frequent family meals were less likely to use tobacco, alcohol, and marijuana. They were also less likely to have a low grade point average or show symptoms of depression. Sitting down for dinner as a family promotes time for relaxation and gives family members a break from an endless list of chores. Moreover, the nutritional benefits of family meals are well proven. Research shows that family dinners are higher in fruits and vegetables, have fewer fried foods, are lower in fat, and have less soda. Children who eat family dinners also tend to have more dairy products at that meal and also are less likely to skip breakfast.

Unsupportive Adults

While a commitment to a healthy-weight home by everyone in the family is ideal, it is not uncommon to have one or more adults in the household be unsupportive. A lack of support or outright sabotage can come from a variety of sources, including a partner, spouse, or caregiver.

Some adults are unwilling to make changes in their own eating or activity behaviors. They may believe that making any changes is not important (for them and/or the child) or they may lack confidence in their ability to succeed, and so they may be unwilling to try.

The lack of support can take a lot of forms. There can be loud complaints that favorite foods are not available or a defiant purchase of those same foods. Noisy objections about limiting screen time or an unwillingness to take part in family-oriented activities may occur. Regardless of how the lack of support is shown, this uncooperative adult, rather than being a role model, makes personal and family decisions that are not helpful.

Unsupportive Spouse or Partner

Parental differences about the creation of a healthy-weight home or any other household matter need to be avoided for the health and well-being of the children. Research finds that children with parents who argue often and intensely are more likely to have problems with their relationship with their parents and have trouble adjusting to uncomfortable situations. Parental conflict can also add to children's feelings of insecurity and inability to cope with problems. Children of divorce are at particular risk when their parents do not get along.

Parents often ask . . .

Which is better, having my kids follow a rule that my spouse won't agree to or not having the rule at all?

Because there are thousands of food and activity behaviors that can be used to create a healthy-weight home, you have the ability to pick and choose. It does not have to be an all-or-nothing battle. Choosing those little changes that your spouse is willing to do and being consistent in following through is generally the recommended strategy.

When it comes to eating, conflicts between parents can have unintentional, harmful results. A high level of family conflict creates stress and the potential for a child to resort to overeating in an effort to deal with the stress. Indeed, research suggests that parents who fight a lot are more likely to have a child who develops an eating disorder.

By contrast, children develop a strong sense of security in their own emotions when parental conflicts are resolved in a positive way. When working toward the creation of a healthy-weight home where the commitment between the parents is different, it is better to compromise and agree to small changes that can be supported by everyone rather than trying to make big changes alone or attempting to force change on someone else.

The amount of change anyone can expect to make depends on his or her role within the family. The parenting that children receive from the one who is most responsible for their care has the greatest effect on the overall change in family structure.

In addition, parenting style makes a difference whether there is conflict between the parents or not. If either parent is authoritarian and overly strict—the enforcer and provider taken to an extreme—there is a risk of turning off the children to the idea of a healthy-weight home and having them rebel against the 5 Simple Rules. However, a parent who is overly permissive or detached—who is not being an enforcer and provider—likewise is not likely to see changes in the children because they have not been guided in how to make wise decisions. The optimal parenting style is *authoritative*—in charge and in control without being overbearing.

Unsupportive Caregivers

In the modern family, there is a strong likelihood that others will help care for our kids. A large number of children live with just one parent. Many have two working parents. Approximately two-thirds of all mothers with children younger than eighteen years work outside the home. Most families with young children depend on caregivers, grandparents, or other adults for childcare. Caregivers can have a big influence on a child's eating and physical activity. What caregivers believe about weight-related habits—their own upbringing, personal food preferences, and other factors—can either help or hinder the creation of a healthy-weight home.

During the time a caregiver is responsible for a child, he or she takes on some or all of the five parenting roles needed to implement the 5 Simple Rules. Caregivers have the power to influence the eating and activity behaviors of children. Research suggests that persuading a child's caregiver to be a food role model results in the child's eating more fruits, vegetables, and dairy products. The caregiver's style is also important. An authoritative feeding style works to get kids to eat more wholesome, nutritious foods. In contrast, an authoritarian feeding style has negative effects, especially on vegetable eating.

Parents often ask . . .

How can I approach my caregiver about what I want?

The best approach is to be direct and give specific instructions. "I don't want the kids to watch too much television" is a vague statement. It is better to say, "The kids can watch television from eight p.m. to nine p.m. and then they need to go to bed." Likewise, expecting the caregiver to create wholesome meals and snacks without direction generally does not work. A better approach is to provide directions about what is to be eaten and when it is to be eaten. For example, "Please give the kids a bowl of cereal with milk at three p.m. and make sure that they eat it at the kitchen table." As a means to reinforce what you want, writing down the instructions also helps.

An open and honest talk with caregivers about the 5 Simple Rules and the way they are being used in the household is an important step in creating a healthy-weight home. Consistency is key. When all the adults who are part of the household are working toward a common goal in a similar way, everyone benefits.

The Importance of Keeping Yourself Healthy

Our own health and well-being affects how well a child adjusts to change in the family structure. Taking care of ourselves is one of the best things that we can do for our kids as well as ourselves. That means being on the lookout for and, if indicated, seeking medical treatment for depression and social withdrawal. Both of these conditions are common in adults going through the death of a loved one, separation, or divorce. A problem that exists and is not dealt with effectively is likely to have a poor impact on the children. Studies suggest that daughters are particularly at risk for developing weight issues when their mothers are depressed.

One of the best things we can do to stay healthy ourselves is to follow the 5 Simple Rules on a daily basis, whether the kids are home or not. If overweight or obesity is an issue, joining a structured weight-loss program and achieving a healthy body weight can help. Research shows that adults who have lost weight with Weight Watchers have a higher quality of life, including less fatigue and enhanced feelings of vigor and vitality.

Chapter 15

When and Where to Get Extra Help

The 5 Simple Rules are the backbone of a healthy-weight home, and the families that live by them will make progress toward a healthy weight. No one can do it alone, though—we need help from schools, communities, and, in some cases, specialists in weight-related fields. While it is beyond this book to provide specific advice about when an expert is needed, this chapter provides some general information about the places that support the principles behind a healthy-weight home, the experts who can provide extra help, and the current recommendations on the use of medications and surgery in kids.

School Support

Schools are a terrific source of support. Because children spend so much time at school, the adults who work in the education system get to know a lot about them. Schools reach children on two levels, in the large groups found in classrooms and in one-on-one contacts. Both lessons in the classroom and individual contacts with supportive teachers can help families who are working toward a healthy weight.

Schools reinforce, both directly and indirectly, the 5 Simple Rules. Many preschools teach simple concepts like healthy snacks and playground games. One study found that going to preschool lowers a child's risk of becoming overweight during the elementary school years. In elementary school, a combination of school and peer support helps kids eat well and be active, leading to less body fat. As children get older, they become both more interested in and sensitive to learning about food and body weight. A weight-education program in ten middle schools helped prevent both weight gain and cut down on disordered eating. Research shows that after-school programs also have a place in preventing overweight in children.

Individual support provided to a child by a school needs to be done in a careful and sensitive way. Successful strategies work by helping the student lose weight in a way that supports the 5 Simple Rules. Working together with schools ensures that any assistance provided is thoughtful, helpful, and done in an empathetic and caring way.

Community Support

As with schools, communities and their organizations can be sources of support and education. One of the strongest predictors of lasting weight loss in adults is having a supportive environment. Community-based weight-gain prevention and education programs for kids tend to be different from those done in the schools. They are designed to build on the school's efforts by giving a fresh point of view using different strategies and goals. Programs in the community are often sponsored by the town's parks or recreation department, the local community center, the Y, houses of worship, sports leagues, service organizations, and dozens of other local organizations.

Professional Resources

Health care professionals can be a valuable source of extra help. Professionals give the specialized advice and treatment families sometimes need to treat a specific weight-related medical or health concern. It helps to have an ongoing relationship with a pediatrician or family physician about weight-related efforts and to proactively bring up any concerns. The pediatrician or family physician is often in the best position to know when a family needs extra help and can refer the family to the right health professional to address special needs. Following is a discussion of some of the health care professionals who work in weight-related specialties, their area of expertise, and the qualifications to consider in seeking professional help.

Registered Dietitians

A registered dietitian (RD) is a food and nutrition expert who completed the college degrees and professional training required by the American Dietetic Association (ADA) to qualify for the credential RD. Dietitians can become certified in either adult or child weight management by completing additional coursework and testing through the ADA. Besides the ADA's RD credentialing, many states license or certify dietitians and nutrition practitioners.

An RD works with the family to develop eating plans that fit its nutrition needs, food preferences, schedule, lifestyle, and medical problems. After an initial evaluation, the RD may continue to work with a family for a period of several months. Many insurance plans cover the services of an RD or include RDs in their network of approved providers.

Dietitians who specialize in weight management work in different types of settings, including hospitals, HMOs, medical groups, doctors' offices, and private practice. They can be located through the ADA's Member Service Center at 1-800-877-1600, ext. 5000, or through the association's Web site at www.eatright.org. Pediatricians and family physicians may be able to recommend a specific RD to a family who needs some extra help.

Certified Physical Trainers or Fitness Professionals

A certified physical trainer or fitness professional is certified in fitness training. Two organizations that provide certification are American Fitness Professionals and Associates (AFPA) and the American Council on

Exercise (ACE). The AFPA has twenty-two different classifications, including personal trainer, aquatics instructor, and children's fitness specialist. The ACE offers four different certifications: personal trainer, group fitness instructor, lifestyle and weight management, and clinical exercise specialist.

Certified fitness professionals work in athletic facilities or gyms, Ys, community centers, and private fitness centers. They can help a family explore activity options and help kids learn how to do activities and exercises correctly to avoid injury.

Local fitness facilities may have qualified trainers on staff. Trainers also advertise in the yellow pages, in local newspapers, and online. Contact information for certified physical trainers and fitness professionals is listed on the AFPA Web site, www.afpafitness.com, at www.acefitness.org, and on the Web site for IDEA Health and Fitness Association at www.ideafit.com.

Psychologists

A licensed clinical or a licensed social psychologist has completed an advanced degree in psychology and passed a psychology board examination, and has a license to practice psychology. Psychologists can help identify behaviors and thoughts that are barriers to achieving a healthy weight and assist in the creation of goals and strategies for change. Psychologists also treat eating disorders. Like RDs, licensed psychologists work in a variety of settings, including hospitals, HMOs, private practice groups, and individual private practices.

Psychologists who specialize in childhood weight issues have experience working with both individual kids and families. They may have received additional training and certifications in eating disorders or child weight management from a medical education program at a university.

A child's pediatrician or the school's psychologist is usually the best source for finding a local psychologist who specializes in childhood weight issues including eating disorders. Other referral sources include the school health department, health clubs or fitness centers, the yellow pages, and the Internet. The American Psychological Association (APA) does not provide direct referrals, but can direct callers to the referral services of state psychological associations. The APA referral number is 1-800-964-2000.

Online Resources

The Internet offers easy access to resources for information, publications, strategies, and other useful information and tips for creating a healthy-weight home. The following are a few of the most reputable sites, along with the topics covered and the types of resources offered:

Fact sheets

American Obesity Association

www.obesity.org

> Fact sheets and information on obesity, its treatment, and prevention

Fitness

Fit Family, Fit Kids

www.verbparents.com

> Articles, tips, and an activity finder to locate regional fitness and activity options

President's Council on Fitness and Sports

www.fitness.gov

> Health, physical activity, sports, and fitness information

Health and weight topics

KidsGrowth Child Health

www.kidsgrowth.com

> Parenting resources, tips, tools, and articles

Weight Watchers International
www.weightwatchers.com
Articles, tools, and recipes for weight management
www.weightwatchers.com/science
Science Center for reliable science information on weight-related topics

Weight-Control Information Network
http://win.niddk.nih.gov/index.htm
Publications on nutrition, physical activity, and weight control

School strategies

Centers for Disease Control and Prevention (CDC) National Center for Chronic Disease Prevention and Health Promotion

Healthy Schools Healthy Youth!
www.cdc.gov/HealthyYouth/index.htm
Publications and strategies for healthy food and physical activity in schools

Mainly for kids

International Food Information Council Foundation
www.kidnetic.com
Games and fitness challenges for children nine to twelve years of age; information pages for parents

TeenGrowth
www.teengrowth.com
Health and weight tips, topics, and discussions especially for teens

Verb
www.verbnow.com
CDC's activity-themed Web site for children

Adult Treatments and Children

The medical community is currently actively debating whether intense adult-based weight-loss treatments like medication or surgery are right for kids. This topic is highly controversial and there is no consensus among health and professional organizations. What is agreed on by experts, however, is that adult treatments should be considered only after a child has a complete workup by a respected pediatric obesity team that has a proven track record and a lot of experience. Professional guidelines are available to help physicians make decisions about treating an overweight child with a treatment designed for adults.

The following is a brief summary of guidelines, recommendations, and regulations about the use of prescription drugs and surgery to treat childhood obesity.

Prescription Drugs

Xenical (orlistat) is the only prescription weight-loss medication approved in the United States for use in teens. It was approved for adolescent use in December 2003. At a dose of 120 mg, orlistat prevents about 30% of the fat in the diet from being digested and absorbed. Because orlistat affects the body's ability to absorb fat-soluble vitamins (A, D, E, and K), it needs to be taken with a daily multivitamin supplement. Orlistat also needs to be combined with behavioral changes that include diet and activity like those in the 5 Simple Rules. One side effect of orlistat, especially if it is not used properly, is oily, fatty stools.

A second medication, Meridia (sibutramine), has been tested overseas on teens but is approved in the United States only for adults. Sibutramine works on the brain's chemistry to reduce appetite, and it also has a minor calorie-burning effect. The side effects of sibutramine include a rise in blood pressure and a faster heart rate.

Surgery

Some physicians consider stomach or intestinal surgery (referred to as bariatric surgery) for extremely obese adolescents (BMI > 40) who also have weight-related medical complications like sleep apnea (poor sleep from interrupted breathing) and type 2 diabetes. There are also exceptions made for teens with a BMI > 50 who have less severe medical problems. It is the position of the European Childhood Obesity Group, a group of experts charged with making recommendations about the medical treatment for overweight children, that surgery should be done only on a very limited basis until studies that look at its safety and long-term effects are known.

Sources

List of Abbreviations

Addict Behav	Addictive Behaviors
Am Fam Physician	American Family Physician
Am J Clin Nutr	American Journal of Clinical Nutrition
Am J Health Behav	American Journal of Health Behavior
Am J Health Promot	American Journal of Health Promotion
Am J Hum Biol	American Journal of Human Biology
Am J Occup Ther	American Journal of Occupational Therapy
Annu Rev Nutr	Annual Review of Nutrition
Annu Rev Public Health	Annual Review of Public Health
Appetite	Appetite
Arch Fam Med	Archives of Family Medicine
Arch Inter Med	Archives of Internal Medicine
Arch Pediatr Adolesc Med	Archives of Pediatric and Adolescent Medicine
Behav Genet	Behavior Genetics
BMJ	British Medical Journal
Bull NY Acad Med	Bulletin of the New York Academy of Medicine
Can J Diet Pract Res	Canadian Journal of Dietetic Practice and Research
Child Adolesc Psychiatr Clin N Am	Child and Adolescent Psychiatric Clinics of North America

Child Care Health Dev	Child: Care, Health and Development
Child Dev	Child Development
Circulation	Circulation
Clin Child Fam Psychol Rev	Clinical Child and Family Psychology Review
Clin Dermatol	Clinical Dermatology
Clin J Sport Med	Clinical Journal of Sport Medicine
Clin Physiol Funct Imaging	Clinical Physiology and Functional Imaging
Crit Rev Food Sci Nutr	CRC Critical Reviews in Food Science and Nutrition
Diabetes Metab	Diabetes & Metabolism
Ethn Dis	Ethnicity & Disease
Ethn Health	Ethnicity & Health
Eval Health Prof	Evaluation & the Health Professions
Health Educ Behav	Health Education & Behavior
Health Psychol	Health Psychology
Health Rep	Health Reports / Statistics Canada
Int J Obes	International Journal of Obesity
Int J Obes Relat Metab Disord	International Journal of Obesity and Related Metabolic Disorders
Int J Paediatr Dent	International Journal of Paediatric Dentistry
Issue Brief Health Policy Track Serv	Issue Brief (Health Policy Tracking Service)
JAMA	Journal of the American Medical Association
J Adolesc Health	Journal of Adolescent Health
J Am Coll Nutr	Journal of the American College of Nutrition
J Am Diet Assoc	Journal of the American Dietetic Association
J Behav Med	Journal of Behavioral Medicine
J Child Adolesc Psychiatr Nurs	Journal of Child and Adolescent Psychiatric Nursing
J Community Health Nurs	Journal of Community Health Nursing

J Consult Clin Psychol	Journal of Consulting and Clinical Psychology
J Fam Psychol	Journal of Family Psychology
J La State Med Soc	Journal of the Louisiana State Medical Society
J Marriage Fam	Journal of Marriage and the Family
J Midwifery Womens Health	Journal of Midwifery & Women's Health
J Nutr Educ	Journal of Nutrition Education
J Nutr Educ Behav	Journal of Nutrition Education and Behavior
J Pediatr	Journal of Pediatrics
J Pediatr Adolesc Gynecol	Journal of Pediatric and Adolescent Gynecology
J Pediatr Psychol	Journal of Pediatric Psychology
J Public Health	Journal of Public Health
J R Soc Health	Journal of the Royal Society of Health
J School Health	Journal of School Health
J Sport Exerc Psychol	Journal of Sport and Exercise Psychology
Lancet	The Lancet
Med J Aust	Medical Journal of Australia
Med Sci Sports Exerc	Medicine and Science in Sports and Exercise
Mil Med	Military Medicine
Minerva Pediatr	Minerva Pediatrica
N Engl J Med	New England Journal of Medicine
Nurs Res	Nursing Research
Obes Res	Obesity Research
Obes Rev	Obesity Reviews
Pediatr Ann	Pediatric Annals
Pediatr Clin North Am	Pediatric Clinics of North America
Pediatr Exer Sci	Pediatric Exercise Science
Pediatr Int	Pediatrics International
Pediatr Nurs	Pediatric Nursing
Pediatrician	Pediatrician
Pediatrics	Pediatrics

Pharmacotherapy	Pharmacotherapy
Physiol Behav	Physiology & Behavior
Phys Med Rehabil Clin N Am	Physical Medicine and Rehabilitation Clinics of North America
Prev Med	Preventive Medicine
Proc Nutr Soc	The Proceedings of the Nutrition Society
Public Health Nutr	Public Health Nutrition
Res Nurs Health	Research in Nursing & Health
Res Q Exerc Sport	Research Quarterly for Exercise and Sport
Rev Endocr Metab Disord	Reviews in Endocrine & Metabolic Disorders
Soc Sci Med	Social Science & Medicine
Surg Obes Rel Dis	Surgery for Obesity and Related Diseases
Women Health	Women & Health

Part One: Introduction

Flodmark C-E, Lissau I, Moreno LA, Pietrobelli A, Widhalm K. New insights into the field of children and adolescents' obesity. *Int J Obes*. 2004; 28:1189–96.

Institute of Medicine of the National Academies. *Preventing Childhood Obesity: Health in the Balance*. Washington, DC: The National Academies Press, 2005.

Iwata F, Hara M, Okada T, Harada K, Li S. Body fat ratios in urban Chinese children. *Pediatr Int*. 2003;45:190–2.

Lissau I, Overpeck MD, Ruan WJ, Due P, Holstein BE, Hediger ML. Health Behaviour in School-Aged Children Obesity Working Group. Body mass index and overweight in adolescents in 13 European countries, Israel, and the United States. *Arch Pediatr Adolesc Med*. 2004;158:27–33.

Ogden CL, Flegal KM, Carroll MD, Johnson CL. Prevalence and trends in overweight among US children and adolescents, 1999–2000. *JAMA*. 2002;288:1728–32.

Prevalence of Overweight among Children and Adolescents: United States, 1999–2002. Centers for Disease Control and Prevention, National Center

for Health Statistics. Accessed online May 4, 2005, at www.cdc.gov/
nchs/products/pubs/pubd/hestats/overwght99.htm.

Chapter 1: When Weight Is an Issue

Barlow S, Dietz W. Obesity evaluation and treatment: Expert committee recommendations. *Pediatrics*. 1998;102(3). Accessed online April 14, 2005, at
www.pediatrics.org/cgi/content/full/102/3/e29.

Centers for Disease Control and Prevention. *BMI—Body Mass Index: BMI for
Children and Teens*. Accessed online May 4, 2005, at www.cdc.gov/
nccdphp/dnpa/bmi/bmi-for-age.htm.

Daniels SR, Arnett DK, Eckel RH, Gidding SS, Hayman LL, Kumanyika S,
Robinson TN, Scott BJ, St Jeor S, Williams CL. Overweight in children and
adolescents: pathophysiology, consequences, prevention, and treatment.
Circulation. 2005;111:1999–2012.

Epstein LH, Valoski AM, Kalarchian MA, McCurley J. Do children lose and
maintain weight easier than adults: a comparison of child and parent weight
changes from six months to ten years. *Obes Res*. 1995;3:411–7.

Epstein LH, Valoski A, Wing RR, McCurley J. Ten-year outcomes of behavioral family-based treatment for childhood obesity. *Health Psychol*.
1994;13:371–2.

Fowler-Brown A, Kahwati LC. Prevention and treatment of overweight in children and adolescents. *Am Fam Physician*. 2004;69:2591–8.

Kleinman RE, ed. *Pediatric Nutrition Handbook,* 5th ed. Chicago: American
Academy of Pediatrics, 2004.

Mueller WH. The changes with age of the anatomical distribution of fat. *Soc
Sci Med*. 1982;16:191–6.

Must A, Jacques PF, Dallal GE, Bajema CJ, Dietz WH. Long-term
morbidity and mortality of overweight adolescents: a follow-up of
the Harvard Growth Study of 1922 to 1935. *N Engl J Med*. 1992;
327:1350–5.

Narayan KM, Boyle JP, Thompson TJ, Sorensen SW, Williamson DF.
Lifetime risk for diabetes mellitus in the United States. *JAMA*.
2003;290:1884–90.

National Task Force on the Prevention and Treatment of Obesity. Overweight, obesity, and health risk. *Arch Intern Med*. 2000;160:898–904.

*Prevalence of Overweight among Children and Adolescents: United States,
1999–2002*. Centers for Disease Control and Prevention, National Center

for Health Statistics. Accessed online May 4, 2005, at www.cdc
.gov/nchs/products/pubs/pubd/hestats/overwght99.htm.

Schwartz MB, Puhl R. Childhood obesity: a societal problem to solve. *Obes Rev.* 2003;4:57–71.

Williams CL, Strobino BA, Bollella M, Brotanek J. Cardiovascular risk reduction in preschool children: the "Healthy Start" project. *J Am Coll Nutr.* 2004;23:117–23.

Chapter 2: Getting Ready for Change

Prochaska JO, Velicer WF. The transtheoretical model of health behavior change. *Am J Health Promot.* 1997;12:38–48.

Velicer WF, Rossi JS, DiClemente CC, Prochaska JO. A criterion measurement model for health behavior change. *Addict Behav.* 1996;21:555–84.

Chapter 3: Kids Are Not Little Adults

Chatterjee N, Blakely DE, Barton C. Perspectives on obesity and barriers to control from workers at a community center serving low-income Hispanic children and families. J *Community Health Nurs.* 2005;22:23–36.

Clarke WR, Lauer RM. Does childhood obesity track into adulthood? *Crit Rev Food Sci Nutr.* 1993;33:423–30.

Epstein LH. Family-based behavioural intervention for obese children. *Int J Obes Relat Metab Disord.* 1996;20:S14–21.

Institute of Medicine of the National Academies. *Preventing Childhood Obesity: Health in the Balance.* Washington, DC: The National Academies Press, 2005.

McLean N, Griffin S, Toney K, Hardeman W. Family involvement in weight control, weight maintenance and weight-loss interventions: a systematic review of randomised trials. *Int J Obes Relat Metab Disord.* 2003; 27:987–1005.

Saxena R, Borzekowski DL, Rickert VI. Physical activity levels among urban adolescent females. *J Pediatr Adolesc Gynecol.* 2002;15:279–84.

Wrotniak BH, Epstein LH, Paluch RA, Roemmich JN. Parent weight change as a predictor of child weight change in family-based behavioral obesity treatment. *Arch Pediatr Adolesc Med.* 2004;158:342–7.

Chapter 4: The 5 Simple Rules

2005 Dietary Guidelines Advisory Committee Report. Accessed online August 8, 2005, at www.health.gov/dietaryguidelines/dga2005/report/.

American Academy of Pediatrics. Policy Statement. Prevention of pediatric overweight and obesity. *Pediatrics*. 2003;112:424–30. Accessed online April 14, 2005, at www.pediatrics.org.

Anderson RE, Crespo CJ, Bartlett SJ, Cheskin LJ, Pratt M. Relationship of physical activity and television watching with body weight and level of fatness among children: results from the Third National Health and Nutrition Examination Survey. *JAMA*. 1998;279:938–42.

Berkey CS, Rockett HR, Gillman MW, Colditz GA. One-year changes in activity and in inactivity among 10- to 15-year-old boys and girls: relationship to change in body mass index. *Pediatrics*. 2003;111: 836–43.

Biddle S, Sallis JF, Cavill NA. *Young and Active? Young People and Health Enhancing Physical Activity. Evidence and Implication*. London: Health Education Authority, 1998.

Birch LL, Davison KK. Family environmental factors influencing the developing behavioral controls of food intake and childhood overweight. *Pediatr Clin North Am*. 2001;48:893–907.

Bowman SA. Beverage choices of young females: changes and impact on nutrient intakes. *J Am Diet Assoc*. 2002;102:1234–9.

Cavill NA, Biddle S, Sallis JF. Health enhancing physical activity for young people: statement of the United Kingdom Expert Consensus Conference. *Pediatric Exer Sci*. 2001;13:12–25.

Clauss SB, Kwiterovich PO. Long-term safety and efficacy of low-fat diets in children and adolescents. *Minerva Pediatr*. 2002;54:305–13.

Deckelbaum RJ, Williams CL. Childhood obesity: the health issue. *Obes Res*. 2001;9:S239–43.

Dennison BA, Erb TA, Jenkins PL. Television viewing and television in bedroom associated with overweight risk among low-income preschool children. *Pediatrics*. 2002;109:1028–35.

Drewnowski A. Taste preferences and food intake. *Ann Rev Nutr*. 1997; 17:237–53.

Edwards CA, Parrett AM. Dietary fibre in infancy and childhood. *Proc Nutr Soc*. 2003;62:17–23.

Field AE, Gillman MW, Rosner B, Rockett HR, Colditz GA. Associations between fruit and vegetable intake and change in body mass index among a large sample of children and adolescents in the United States. *Int J Obes*. 2003;27:821–6.

Gillman MW, Rifas-Shiman SL, Frazier AL, Rockett HR, Camargo CA Jr, Field AE, Berkey CS, Colditz GA. Family dinner and diet quality among older children and adolescents. *Arch Fam Med.* 2000;9:235–40.

Golan M, Weizman A. Familial approach to the treatment of childhood obesity: conceptual mode. *J Nutr Educ.* 2001;33:102–7.

Hancox RJ, Milne BJ, Poulton R. Association between child and adolescent television viewing and adult health: a longitudinal birth cohort study. *Lancet.* 2004;364:257–62.

Harnack L, Stang J, Story M. Soft drink consumption among US children and adolescents: nutritional consequences. *J Am Diet Assoc.* 1999;99:436–41.

James J, Thomas P, Cavan D, Kerr D. Preventing childhood obesity by reducing consumption of carbonated drinks: cluster randomised controlled trial. *BMJ.* 2004;328:1237. Epub 2004 Apr 23.

Levin S, Lowry R, Brown DR, Dietz WH. Physical activity and body mass index among US adolescents. *Arch Pediatr Adolesc Med.* 2003;157:816–20.

Nicklas T, Johnson R; American Dietetic Association. Position of the American Dietetic Association: dietary guidance for healthy children ages 2 to 11 years. *J Am Diet Assoc.* 2004;104:660–77.

Orlet Fisher J, Rolls BJ, Birch LL. Children's bite size and intake of an entree are greater with large portions than with age-appropriate or self-selected portions. *Am J Clin Nutr.* 2003;77:1164–70.

Physical Activity and Health: A Report of the Surgeon General. Atlanta, GA: US Department of Health and Human Services, Centers for Disease Control and Prevention, National Center for Chronic Disease Prevention and Health Promotion, 1996.

Rajeshwari R, Yang SJ, Nicklas TA, Berenson GS. Secular trends in children's sweetened-beverage consumption (1973 to 1994): the Bogalusa Heart Study. *J Am Diet Assoc.* 2005;105:208–14.

Rampersaud GC, Pereira MA, Girard BL, Adams J, Metzl JD. Breakfast habits, nutritional status, body weight, and academic performance in children and adolescents. *J Am Diet Assoc.* 2005;105:743–60.

Ritchie LD, Welk G, Styne D, Gerstein DE, Crawford PB. Family environment and pediatric overweight: what is a parent to do? *J Am Diet Assoc.* 2005;105:S70–9.

Rolls BJ, Engell D, Birch LL. Serving portion size influences 5-year-old but not 3-year-old children's food intakes. *J Am Diet Assoc.* 2000;100:232–4.

St.-Onge MP, Keller KL, Heymsfield SB. Changes in childhood food consumption patterns: a cause for concern in light of increasing body weights. *Am J Clin Nutr*. 2003;78:1068–73.

Williams CL, Hayman LL, Daniels SR, Robinson TN, Steinberger J, Paridon S, Bazzarre T. Cardiovascular health in childhood: a statement for health professionals from the Committee on Atherosclerosis, Hypertension, and Obesity in the Young (AHOY) of the Council on Cardiovascular Disease in the Young, American Heart Association. *Circulation*. 2002;106:143–60.

Wyatt HR, Grunwald GK, Mosca CL, Klem ML, Wing RR, Hill JO. Long-term weight loss and breakfast in subjects in the National Weight Control Registry. *Obes Res*. 2002;10:78–82.

Young LR, Nestle M. The contribution of expanding portion sizes to the US obesity epidemic. *Am J Public Health*. 2002;92:246–9.

Young LR, Nestle M. Expanding portion sizes in the US marketplace: implications for nutrition counseling. *J Am Diet Assoc*. 2003;103:231–4.

Chapter 5: The Roles Parents Play

Adams Larsen M, Tentis E. The art and science of disciplining children. *Pediatr Clin North Am*. 2003;50:817–40.

American Academy of Pediatrics. Family pediatrics: report of the Task Force on the Family. *Pediatrics*. 2003;1541–71. Accessed online April 30, 2005, at www.pediatrics.org/cgi/content/full/111/6/S1/1541.

American Heritage Dictionary of the English Language, 4th ed. New York: Houghton Mifflin Company, 2003.

Barlow J, Underdown A. Promoting the social and emotional health of children: where to now? *J R Soc Health*. 2005;125:64–70.

Barlow SE, Dietz W Jr. Obesity evaluation and treatment: expert committee recommendations. *Pediatrics*. 1998;102:e29.

Birch LL. Development of food acceptance patterns in the first years of life. *Proc Nutr* Soc. 1998;57:617–24.

Birch LL, Davison KK. Family environmental factors influencing the developing behavioral controls of food intake and childhood overweight. *Ped Clin N Am*. 2001;48:893–907.

Cathey M, Gaylord N. Picky eating: a toddler's continuing approach to mealtime. *Pediatr Nurs*. 2004;30:101–7.

Fox KR. Childhood obesity and the role of physical activity. *J R Soc Health*. 2004;124:34–9.

Golan M, Weizman A. Familial approach to the treatment of childhood obesity: conceptual mode. *J Nutr Educ*. 2001;33:102–7.

Henze C, Plaza CI. Public health issue brief: physical education: year end report—2004. *Issue Brief Health Policy Track Serv*. 2004;1–16.

Hertzler AA. Children's food patterns—a review: II. Family and group behavior. *J Am Diet Assoc*. 1983;83:555–60.

Hertzler AA. Obesity—impact of the family. *J Am Diet Assoc*. 1981; 79:525–30.

Hood VL, Kelly B, Martinez C, Shuman S, Secker-Walker R. A Native American community initiative to prevent diabetes. *Ethn Health*. 1997;2:277–85.

Kalb LM, Loeber R. Child disobedience and noncompliance: a review. *Pediatrics*. 2003;111:641–52.

Kolliker M. Ontogeny in the family. *Behav Genet*. 2005;35:7–18.

Licence K. Promoting and protecting the health of children and young people. *Child Care Health Dev*. 2004;30:623–35.

Longjohn MM. Chicago project uses ecological approach to obesity prevention. *Pediatr Ann*. 2004;33:55–7, 62–3.

McBean LD, Miller GD. Enhancing the nutrition of America's youth. *J Am Coll Nutr*. 1999;18:563–71.

McCaffree J. Childhood eating patterns: the roles parents play. *J Am Diet Assoc*. 2003;103:1587.

Moore H, Nelson P, Marshall J, Cooper M, Zambas H, Brewster K, Atkin K. Laying foundations for health: food provision for under 5s in day care. *Appetite*. 2005;44:207–13.

Moore LL, Lombardi DA, White MJ, Campbell JL, Oliveria SA, Ellison RC. Influence of parents' physical activity levels on activity levels of young children. *J Pediatr*. 1991;118:215–9.

Position of the American Dietetic Association: benchmarks for nutrition programs in child care settings. *J Am Diet Assoc*. 2005;105:979–86.

Weiss MR, Ebbeck V, Horn TS. Children's self-perceptions and sources of physical competence information: a cluster analysis. *J Sport Exerc Psychol*. 1997;19:52–70.

Chapter 6: The Kids Are Watching

Benton D. Role of parents in the determination of the food preferences of children and the development of obesity. *Int J Obes Relat Metab Disord*. 2004;28:858–69.

Birch LL. Generalization of a modified food preference. *Child Dev.* 1981;52:755–8.

Coon KA, Goldberg J, Rogers BL, Tucker KL. Relationships between use of television during meals and children's food consumption patterns. *Pediatrics.* 2001;107:e7.

Fisher JO, Birch LL. Restricting access to foods and children's eating. *Appetite.* 1999;32:405–19.

Fox MK, Pac S, Devaney B, Jankowski L. Feeding infants and toddlers study: what foods are infants and toddlers eating? *J Am Diet Assoc.* 2004; 104:S22–30.

Gillman MW, Rifas-Shiman SL, Frazier AL, Rockett HR, Camargo CA Jr, Field AE, Berkey CS, Colditz GA. Family dinner and diet quality among older children and adolescents. *Arch Fam Med.* 2000;9:235–40.

Golan M, Crow S. Targeting parents exclusively in the treatment of childhood obesity: long-term results. *Obes Res.* 2004;12:357–61.

Golan M, Weizman A. Familial approach to the treatment of childhood obesity: conceptual mode. *J Nutr Educ.* 2001;33:102–7.

Golan M, Weizman A, Apter A, Fainaru M. Parents as the exclusive agents of change in the treatment of childhood obesity. *Am J Clin Nutr.* 1998; 67:1130–5.

Institute of Medicine of the National Academies. *Preventing Childhood Obesity: Health in the Balance.* Washington, DC: The National Academies Press, 2005.

Johnson SL, McPhee L, Birch LL. Conditioned preferences: young children prefer flavors associated with high dietary fat. *Physiol Behav.* 1991;50:1245–51.

Lederman SA, Akabas SR, Moore BJ, Bentley ME, Devaney B, Gillman MW, Kramer MS, Mennella JA, Ness A, Wardle J. Summary of the presentations at the Conference on Preventing Childhood Obesity, December 8, 2003. *Pediatrics.* 2004;114:1146–73.

McCaffree J. Childhood eating patterns: the roles parents play. *J Am Diet Assoc.* 2003;103:1587.

McConahy KL, Smiciklas-Wright H, Birch LL, Mitchell DC, Picciano MF. Food portions are positively related to energy intake and body weight in early childhood. *J Pediatr.* 2002;140:340–7.

Nicklaus S, Boggio V, Chabanet C, Issanchou S. A prospective study of food variety seeking in childhood, adolescence and early adult life. *Appetite.* 2005;44:289–97.

Orlet Fisher J, Rolls BJ, Birch LL. Children's bite size and intake of an entree are greater with large portions than with age-appropriate or self-selected portions. *Am J Clin Nutr.* 2003;77:1164–70.

Rolls BJ, Engell D, Birch LL. Serving portion size influences 5-year-old but not 3-year-old children's food intakes. *J Am Diet Assoc.* 2000;100:232–4.

Story M, Holt K, Sofka D. *Bright Futures in Practice: Nutrition*, 2nd ed. Arlington, VA: National Center for Education in Maternal and Child Health, 2002.

Sullivan SA, Birch LL. Infant dietary experience and acceptance of solid foods. *Pediatrics.* 1994;93:271–7.

Whitaker RC, Wright JA, Pepe MS, Seidel KD, Dietz WH. Predicting obesity in young adulthood from childhood and parental obesity. *N Engl J Med.* 1997;337:869–73.

Chapter 7: Active Parents, Active Kids

2005 Dietary Guidelines Advisory Committee Report. Accessed online August 8, 2005, at www.health.gov/dietaryguidelines/dga2005/report/.

American Academy of Pediatrics Committee on Public Education. Children, adolescents, and television. *Pediatrics.* 2001;107:423–6.

Anderssen N, Wold B. Parental and peer influences on leisure-time physical activity in young adolescents. *Res Q Exerc Sport.* 1992;63:341–8.

Bandura A. Self-efficacy: the exercise of control. *Am J Health Promotion.* 1997;12:8–12.

Barlow S, Dietz W. Obesity evaluation and treatment: expert committee recommendations. *Pediatrics.* 1998;102:e29. Accessed online April 14, 2005, at www.pediatrics.org/cgi/content/full/102/3/e29.

Brustad RJ. Who will go out and play? Parental and psychological influences on children's attraction to physical activity. *Pediatric Exercise Science.* 1993;5:210–23.

Chakravarthy MV, Booth FW. Inactivity and inaction. *Arch Pediatr Adolesc Med.* 2003;157:731–2.

Daniels SR, Arnett DK, Eckel RH, Gidding SS, Hayman LL, Kumanyika S, Robinson TN, Scott BJ, St Jeor S, Williams CL. Overweight in children and adolescents: pathophysiology, consequences, prevention, and treatment. *Circulation.* 2005;111:1999–2012.

Davison KK, Cutting TM, Birch LL. Parents' activity-related parenting practices predict girls' physical activity. *Med Sci Sports Exerc.* 2003; 35:1589–95.

DiLorenzo TM, Stucky-Ropp RC, Vander Wal JS, Gotham HJ. Determinants of exercise among children. II. A longitudinal analysis. *Prev Med.* 1998;27:470–7.

Freedson PS, Evenson S. Familial aggregation in physical activity. *Res Q Exerc Sport.* 1991;62:384–9.

Gutin B, Yin Z, Humphries MC, Barbeau P. Relations of moderate and vigorous physical activity to fitness and fatness in adolescents. *Am J Clin Nutr.* 2005;81:746–50.

Healthy People 2010. Accessed online May 11, 2005, at www.healthy people.gov.

Institute of Medicine of the National Academies. *Preventing Childhood Obesity: Health in the Balance.* Washington, DC: The National Academies Press, 2005.

Kalakanis LE, Goldfield GS, Paluch RA, Epstein LH. Parental activity as a determinant of activity level and patterns of activity in obese children. *Res Q Exerc Sport.* 2001;72:202–9.

Kohl HW, Hobbs KE. Development of physical activity behaviors among children and adolescents. *Pediatrics.* 1998;101:549–54.

Moore LL, Lombardi DA, White MJ, Campbell JL, Olshan AF, Ellison RC. Influence of parents physical activity levels on activity levels of young children. *Pediatrics.* 1991;118:215–9.

Patrick K, Spear B, Holt K, Sofka D, Eds. *Bright Futures in Practice: Physical Activity.* Arlington, VA: National Center for Education in Maternal and Child Health, 2001.

Scanlan TK, Simons JP. The construct of sports enjoyment. In Roberts GC (Ed.). *Motivation in Sport and Exercise.* Champaign, IL: Human Kinetics, 1992.

Stucky-Ropp RC, DiLorenzo TM. Determinants of exercise in children. *Prev Med.* 1993;22:880–9.

U.S Surgeon General. *The Surgeon General's Call to Action to Prevent and Decrease Overweight and Obesity.* Accessed online August 8, 2005, at www.surgeongeneral.gov/topics/obesity/calltoaction/.

Weight-Control Information Network. Accessed online May 11, 2005, at http://win.niddk.nih.gov/index.htm.

Weiss, MR. Motivating kids in physical activity. *President's Council on Physical Fitness and Sports Research Digest.* September 2000;3(11).

Welk GJ. *Promoting Physical Activity in Children: Parental Influences*. Washington, DC: ERIC Clearinghouse on Teaching and Teacher Education, 2000. Accessed online May 11, 2005, at www.ericdigests.org/2000-3/activity.htm.

Whitaker RC. Obesity prevention in pediatric primary care. *Arch Pediatr Adolesc Med*. 2003;157:725–7.

Writing Group. Understanding obesity in youth. *Circulation*. 1996;94:3383–7.

Chapter 8: Putting Food on the Table

Barlow SE, Dietz W Jr. Obesity evaluation and treatment: expert committee recommendations. *Pediatrics*. 1998;102:e29.

Birch LL, Davison KK. Family environmental factors influencing the developing behavioral controls of food intake and childhood overweight. *Pediatr Clin North Am*. 2001;48:893–907.

Birch LL, Deysher M. Caloric compensation and sensory specific satiety: evidence for self regulation of food intake by young children. *Appetite*. 1986;7:323–31.

Birch LL, Fisher JO. Development of eating behaviors among children and adolescents. *Pediatrics*. 1998;101:539–49.

Birch LL, Marlin D, Rotter J. Eating as the "means" activity in a contingency: effects on young children's food preference. *Child Dev*. 1984;55:532–9.

Birch LL, Zimmerman S, Hind H. The influence of social affective context on preschool children's food preferences. *Child Dev*. 1980;51:856–61.

Committee on Nutrition. Prevention of pediatric overweight and obesity. *Pediatrics*. 2003;112:424–30.

Cullen KW, Baranowski T, Owens E, Marsh T, Rittenberry L, de Moor C. Availability, accessibility, and preferences for fruit, 100% fruit juice, and vegetables influence children's dietary behavior. *Health Educ Behav*. 2003;30:615–26.

Ebbeling CB, Sinclair KB, Pereira MA, Garcia-Lago E, Feldman HA, Ludwig DS. Compensation for energy intake from fast food among overweight and lean adolescents. *JAMA*. 2004;291:2828–33.

Golan M, Crow S. Targeting parents exclusively in the treatment of childhood obesity: long-term results. *Obes Res*. 2004;12:358.

Institute of Medicine of the National Academies. *Preventing Childhood Obesity: Health in the Balance*. Washington, DC: The National Academies Press, 2005.

Johnson SL, McPhee L, Birch LL. Conditioned preferences: young children prefer flavors associated with high dietary fat. *Physiol Behav*. 1991;50:1245–51.

Loewen R, Pliner P. Effects of prior exposure to palatable and unpalatable novel foods on children's willingness to taste other novel foods. *Appetite*. 1999;32:351–66.

Ludwig DS, Peterson KE, Gortmaker SL. Relation between consumption of sugar-sweetened drinks and childhood obesity: a prospective, observational analysis. *Lancet*. 2001;357:505–8.

Pliner P, Loewen R. The effects of manipulated arousal on children's willingness to taste novel foods. *Physiol Behav*. 2002;76:551–8.

Sullivan SA, Birch LL. Infant dietary experience and acceptance of solid foods. *Pediatrics*. 1994;93:271–7.

Chapter 9: Helping Kids Move

Anderssen N, Wold B. Parental and peer influences on leisure-time physical activity in young adolescents. *Res Q Exerc Sport*. 1992;63:341–8.

Biddle S. Goudas, M. Analysis of children's physical activity and its association with adult encouragement and social cognitive values. *J School Health*. 1996;66:75–8.

Brustad RJ. Parental and peer influence on children's psychological development through sport. In Smoll FL, Smith RE (Eds.). *Children and Youth in Sport: A Biopsychosocial Perspective*. Madison, WI: Brown and Benchmark, 1996.

Brustad RJ. Who will go out and play? Parental and psychological influences on children's attraction to physical activity. *Pediatr Exer Sci*. 1993;5:210–23.

Craig S, Goldberg J, Dietz WH. Psychosocial correlates of physical activity among fifth and eighth graders. *Prev Med*. 1996;25:506–13.

Daniels SR, Arnett DK, Eckel RH, Gidding SS, Hayman LL, Kumanyika S, Robinson TN, Scott BJ, St. Jeor S, Williams CL. Overweight in children and adolescents. *Circulation*. 2005;11:1999–2012.

Fowler-Brown A, Kahwati LC. Prevention and treatment of overweight in children and adolescents. *Am Fam Physician*. 2004;69:2591–8.

Gortmaker SL, Must A, Sobol AM, Peterson K, Colditz GA, Dietz WH. Television viewing as a cause of increasing obesity among children in the United States, 1986–1990. *Arch Pediatr Adolesc Med*. 1996; 150:356–62.

Institute of Medicine of the National Academies. *Preventing Childhood Obesity: Health in the Balance.* Washington, DC: The National Academies Press, 2005.

Kimiecik JC, Horn TS, Shurin CS. Relationships among children's beliefs, perceptions of their parents' beliefs, and their moderate-to-vigorous physical activity. *Res Q Exer Sport.* 1966;67:324–36.

McGuire MT, Hannan PJ, Neumark-Sztainer D, Cossrow NH, Story M. Parental correlates of physical activity in a racially/ethnically diverse adolescent sample. *J Adolesc Health.* 2002;30:253–61.

McKenzie TL, Li D, Derby CA, Webber LS, Luepker RV, Cribb P. Maintenance of effects of the CATCH physical education program: results from the CATCH-ON study. *Health Educ Behav.* 2003;30:447–62.

Sallis JF, Prochaska JJ, Taylor WC. A review of correlates of physical activity of children and adolescents. *Med Sci Sports Exerc.* 2000;32:963–75.

Shape Up America! Accessed online May 24, 2005, at www.shapeup america.org.

U.S Surgeon General. *The Surgeon General's Call to Action to Prevent and Decrease Overweight and Obesity.* Accessed online August 8, 2005, at www.surgeongeneral.gov/topics/obesity/calltoaction/.

Weiss MR. Motivating kids in physical activity. *President's Council on Physical Fitness and Sports Research Digest.* September 2000;3(11).

Weiss MR, Ebbeck V. Self-esteem and perceptions of competence in youth sport: theory, research, and enhancement strategies. In Bar-Or O (Ed.). *The Encyclopedia of Sports Medicine, Volume 4: The Child and Adolescent Athlete.* Oxford, UK: Blackwell Science, 1996.

Welk GJ. *Promoting Physical Activity in Children: Parental Influences.* Washington, DC: ERIC Clearinghouse on Teaching and Teacher Education, 1999.

Chapter 10: Setting Food Policy

Birch LL, Davison KK. Family environmental factors influencing the developing behavioral controls of food intake and childhood overweight. *Pediatr Clin North Am.* 2001;48:893–907.

Cooke LJ, Wardle J, Gibson EL, Sapochnik M, Sheiham A, Lawson M. Demographic, familial and trait predictors of fruit and vegetable consumption by pre-school children. *Public Health Nutr.* 2004;7:295–302.

Eisenberg ME, Olson RE, Neumark-Sztainer D, Story M, Bearinger LH. Correlations between family meals and psychosocial well-being among adolescents. *Arch Pediatr Adolesc Med.* 2004;158:792–6.

Granner ML, Sargent RG, Calderon KS, Hussey JR, Evans AE, Watkins KW. Factors of fruit and vegetable intake by race, gender, and age among young adolescents. *J Nutr Educ Behav.* 2004;36:173–80.

Hanson NI, Neumark-Sztainer D, Eisenberg ME, Story M, Wall M. Associations between parental report of the home food environment and adolescent intakes of fruits, vegetables and dairy foods. *Public Health Nutr.* 2005;8:77–85.

Hood MY, Moore LL, Sundarajan-Ramamurti A, Singer M, Cupples LA, Ellison RC. Parental eating attitudes and the development of obesity in children. The Framingham Children's Study. *Int J Obes Relat Metab Disord.* 2000;24:1319–25.

Institute of Medicine of the National Academies. *Preventing Childhood Obesity: Health in the Balance.* Washington, DC: The National Academies Press, 2005.

Johnson SL. Improving preschoolers' self-regulation of energy intake. *Pediatrics.* 2000;106:1429–35.

Kremers SP, Bur J, De Vries H, Engels RC. Parenting style and adolescent fruit consumption. *Appetite.* 2003;42:43–50.

Lande B, Andersen LF, Veierod MB, Baerug A, Johansson L, Trygg KU, Bjorneboe GE. Breast-feeding at 12 months of age and dietary habits among breast-fed and non-breast-fed infants. *Public Health Nutr.* 2004;7:495–503.

Le Bigot Macaux A. Eat to live or live to eat? Do parents and children agree? *Public Health Nutr.* 2001;4:141–6.

Liem DG, Mars M, De Graaf C. Sweet preference and sugar consumption of 4- and 5-year-old children: role of parents. *Appetite.* 2004;43:235–45.

Marquis M, Filion YP, Dagenais F. Does eating while watching television influence children's food-related behaviours? *Can J Diet Pract Res.* 2005;66:12–8.

Neumark-Sztainer D, Wall M, Story M, Fulkerson JA. Are family meal patterns associated with disordered eating behaviors among adolescents? *J Adolesc Health.* 2004;35:350–9.

Roberts BP, Blinkhorn AS, Duxbury JT. The power of children over adults when obtaining sweet snacks. *Int J Paediatr Dent.* 2003;13:76–84.

Shunk JA, Birch LL. Girls at risk for overweight at age 5 are at risk for dietary restraint, disinhibited overeating, weight concerns, and great weight gain from 5 to 9 years. *J Am Diet Assoc.* 2004;104:1120–6.

Stice E, Presnell K, Shaw H, Rohde P. Psychological and behavioral risk factors for obesity onset in adolescent girls: a prospective study. *J Consult Clin Psychol*. 2005;73:195–202.

Videon TM, Manning CK. Influences on adolescent eating patterns: the importance of family meals. *J Adolesc Health*. 2003;32:365–73.

Chapter 11: Sit Less, Move More

Arluk SL, Branch JD, Swain DP, Dowling EA. Childhood obesity's relationship to time spent in sedentary behavior. *Mil Med*. 2003;168:583–6.

Baur LA, O'Connor J. Special considerations in childhood and adolescent obesity. *Clin Dermatol*. 2004;22:338–44.

Brustad RJ. Attraction to physical activity in urban schoolchildren: parental socialization and gender influences. *Res Q Exerc Sport*. 1996;68:316–23.

Craig S, Goldberg J, Dietz WH. Psychosocial correlates of physical activity among fifth and eighth graders. *Prev Med*. 1996;25:506–13.

Davison KK, Birch LL. Obesigenic families: parents' physical activity and dietary intake patterns predict girls' risk of overweight. *Int J Obes Relat Metab Disord*. 2002;26:1186–93.

Davison KK, Cutting TM, Birch LL. Parents' activity-related parenting practices predict girls' physical activity. *Med Sci Sports Exerc*. 2003;35:1589–95.

Dennison BA, Erb TA, Jenkins PL. Television viewing and television in bedroom associated with overweight risk among low-income preschool children. *Pediatrics*. 2002;109:1028–35.

DiLorenzo TM, Stucky-Ropp RC, Vander Wal JS, Gotham HJ. Determinants of exercise among children. II. A longitudinal analysis. *Prev Med*. 1998;27:470–7.

Epstein LH, Paluch RA, Gordy CC, Dorn J. Decreasing sedentary behaviors in treating pediatric obesity. *Arch Pediatr Adolesc Med*. 2000;154:220–6.

Epstein LH, Valoski AM, Vara LS, McCurley J, Wisniewski L, Kalarchian MA, Klein KR, Shrager LF. Effects of decreasing sedentary behavior and increasing activity on weight change in obese children. *Health Psychol*. 1995;14:109–15.

Faith MS, Leone MA, Ayers TS, Heo M, Pietrobelli A. Weight criticism during physical activity, coping skills, and reported physical activity in children. *Pediatrics*. 2002;110:e23.

Fogelholm M, Nuutinen O, Pasanen M, Myohanen E, Saatela T. Parent-child relationship of physical activity patterns and obesity. *Int J Obes Relat Metab Disord.* 1999;23:1262–8.

Golan M, Fainaru M, Weizman A. Role of behaviour modification in the treatment of childhood obesity with the parents as the exclusive agents of change. *Int J Obes Relat Metab Disord.* 1998;22:1217–24.

Golan M, Weizman A. Familial approach to the treatment of childhood obesity: conceptual mode. *J Nutr Educ.* 2001;33:102–7.

Institute of Medicine of the National Academies. *Preventing Childhood Obesity: Health in the Balance.* Washington, DC: The National Academies Press, 2005.

Kimiecik JC, Horn TS. Parental beliefs and children's moderate-to-vigorous physical activity. *Res Q Exerc Sport.* 1998;69:163–75.

Moore LL, Lombardi DA, White MJ, Campbell JL, Oliveria SA, Ellison RC. Influence of parents' physical activity levels on activity levels of young children. *J Pediatr.* 1991;118:215–9.

Perez CE. Children who become active. *Health Rep.* 2003;14 (Suppl):17–28.

Proctor MH, Moore LL, Gao D, Cupples LA, Bradlee ML, Hood MY, Ellison RC. Television viewing and change in body fat from preschool to early adolescence: the Framingham Children's Study. *Int J Obes Relat Disord.* 2003;27:827–33.

Ritchie LD, Welk G, Styne D, Gerstein DE, Crawford PB. Family environment and pediatric overweight: what is a parent to do? *J Am Diet Assoc.* 2005;105:S70–9.

Robinson TN, Killen JD, Kraemer HC, Wilson DM, Matheson DM, Haskell WL, Pruitt LA, Powell TM, Owens AS, Thompson NS, Flint-Moore NM, Davis GJ, Emig KA, Brown RT, Rochon J, Green S, Varady A. Dance and reducing television viewing to prevent weight gain in African-American girls: the Stanford GEMS pilot study. *Ethn Dis.* 2003;13:S65–77.

Sallis JF, McKenzie TL, Elder JP, Broyles SL, Nader PR. Factors parents use in selecting play spaces for young children. *Arch Pediar Adolesc Med.* 1997;151:414–7.

Stucky-Ropp RC, DiLorenzo TM. Determinants of exercise in children. *Prev Med.* 1993;22:880–9.

Trost SG, Pate RR, Saunders R, Ward DS, Dowda M, Felton G. A prospective study of the determinants of physical activity in rural fifth-grade children. *Prev Med.* 1997;26:257–63.

Trost SG, Sallis JF, Pate RR, Freedson PS, Taylor WC, Dowda M. Evaluating a model of parental influence on youth physical activity. *Am J Prev Med.* 2003;25:277–82.

Trost SG, Sirard JR, Dowda M, Pfeiffer KA, Pate RR. Physical activity in overweight and nonoverweight preschool children. *Int J Obes Relat Metab Disord.* 2003;27:834–9.

U.S Surgeon General. *The Surgeon General's Call to Action to Prevent and Decrease Overweight and Obesity.* Accessed online August 8, 2005, at www.surgeongeneral.gov/topics/obesity/calltoaction/.

Wagner A, Klein-Platat C, Arveiler D, Haan MC, Schlienger JL, Simon C. Parent-child physical activity relationships in 12-year old French students do not depend on family socioeconomic status. *Diabetes Metab.* 2004; 30:359–66.

Chapter 12: Being on the Lookout

Bell SK, Morgan SB. Children's attitudes and behavioral intentions toward a peer presented as obese: does a medical explanation for the obesity make a difference? *J Pediatr Psychol.* 2000;25:137–45.

Braet C, Mervielde I, Vandereycken W. Psychological aspects of childhood obesity: a controlled study in a clinical and nonclinical sample. *J Pediatr Psychol.* 1997;22:59–71.

Brehm BJ, Rourke KM, Cassell C, Sethuraman G. Psychosocial outcomes of a pilot multidisciplinary program for weight management. *Am J Health Behav.* 2003;27:348–54.

Family pediatrics: report of the Task Force on the Family. *Pediatrics.* 2003;111:1541–71.

Janssen I, Craig WM, Boyce WF, Pickett W. Associations between overweight and obesity with bullying behaviors in school-aged children. *Pediatrics.* 2004;113:1187–94.

Kramer L, Perozynski LA, Chung TY. Parental responses to sibling conflict: the effects of development and parent gender. *Child Dev.* 1999; 70:1401–14.

Latner JD, Stunkard AJ. Getting worse: the stigmatization of obese children. *Obes Res.* 2003;11:452–6.

Malina RM. Physical activity and fitness: pathways from childhood to adulthood. *Am J Hum Biol.* 2001;13:162–72.

Malina RM. Tracking of physical activity and physical fitness across the lifespan. *Res Q Exerc Sport.* 1996;67:S548–57.

Manus HE, Killeen MR. Maintenance of self-esteem by obese children. *J Child Adolesc Psychiatr Nurs*. 1995;8:17–27.

Marinov B, Kostianev S, Turnovska T. Ventilatory efficiency and rate of perceived exertion in obese and non-obese children performing standardized exercise. *Clin Physiol Funct Imaging*. 2002;22:254–60.

Musher-Eizenman DR, Holub SC, Miller AB, Goldstein SE, Edwards-Leeper L. Body size stigmatization in preschool children: the role of control attributions. *J Pediatr Psychol*. 2004;29:613–20.

Neumark-Sztainer D, Story M, Hannan PJ, Tharp T, Rex J. Factors associated with changes in physical activity: a cohort study of inactive adolescent girls. *Arch Pediatr Adolesc Med*. 2003;157:803–10.

Norman A-C, Drinkard B, McDuffie JR, Ghorbani S, Yanoff YB, Yanovski JA. Influence of excess adiposity on exercise fitness and performance in overweight children and adolescents. *Pediatrics*. 2005;115:e690.

Robbins LB, Pender NJ, Kazanis AS. Barriers to physical activity perceived by adolescent girls. *J Midwifery Womens Health*. 2003;48:203–12.

Schor EL. Developing communality: family-centered programs to improve children's health and well-being. *Bull NY Acad Med*. 1995; 72:413–42.

Strauss RS. Childhood obesity and self-esteem. *Pediatrics*. 2000;105:e15.

Strauss RS, Pollack HA. Social marginalization of overweight children. *Arch Pediatr Adolsc Med*. 2003;157:746–52.

Taylor WC, Yancey AK, Leslie J, Murray NG, Cummings SS, Sharkey SA, Wert C, James J, Miles O, McCarthy WJ. Physical activity among African American and Latino middle school girls: consistent beliefs, expectations, and experiences access two sites. *Women Health*. 1999;30:67–82.

Timm NL, Grupp-Phelan J, Ho ML. Chronic ankle morbidity in obese children following an acute ankle injury. *Arch Pediatr Adolesc Med*. 2005; 159:33–6.

Zabinski MF, Saelens BE, Stein RI, Hayden-Wade HA, Wilfley DE. Overweight children's barriers to and support for physical activity. *Obes Res*. 2003;11:238–46.

Chapter 13: Taking It outside the Home

Barlow SE, Dietz WH. Obesity evaluation and treatment: expert committee recommendations. *Pediatrics*. 1998;102:e29.

Batch JA, Baur LA. Management and prevention of obesity and its complications in children and adolescents. *Med J Aust*. 2005;182:130–5.

Borra ST, Kelly L, Shirreffs MB, Neville K, Geiger CJ. Developing health messages: qualitative studies with children, parents, and teachers help identify communications opportunities for healthful lifestyles and the prevention of obesity. *J Am Diet Assoc*. 2003;103:721–8.

Caballero B. Obesity prevention in children: opportunities and challenges. *Int J Obes Relat Metab Disord*. 2004;28:S90–5.

Carlisle LK, Gordon ST, Sothern MS. Can obesity prevention work for our children? *J La State Med Soc*. 2005;157:S34–41.

Dietz WH, Gortmaker SL. Preventing obesity in children and adolescents. *Annu Rev Public Health*. 2001;22:337–53.

Dietz WH, Robinson TN. Overweight children and adolescents. *N Engl J Med*. 2005;352:2100–9.

Institute of Medicine of the National Academies. *Preventing Childhood Obesity: Health in the Balance*. Washington, DC: The National Academies Press, 2005.

Lissau I, Sorensen TI. Parental neglect during childhood and increased risk of obesity in young adulthood. *Lancet*. 1994;343:324–7.

Lissau I, Sorensen TI. School difficulties in childhood and risk of overweight and obesity in young adulthood: a ten year prospective population study. *Int J Obes Relat Metab Disord*. 1993;17:169–75.

McCaffree J. Childhood eating patterns: the roles parents play. *J Am Diet Assoc*. 2003;103:1587.

Muller MJ, Asbeck I , Mast M, Langnase K, Grund A. Prevention of obesity—more than an intention: concept and first results of the Kiel Obesity Prevention Study (KOPS). *Int J Obes Relat Metab Disord*. 2001;25:S66–74.

Olson CM. Childhood nutrition education in health promotion and disease prevention. *Bull NY Acad Med*. 1989;65:1143–53.

Shephard RJ. Role of the physician in childhood obesity. *Clin J Sport Med*. 2004;14:161–8.

Williams CL. Nutrition intervention and health risk reduction in childhood: creating healthy adults. *Pediatrician*. 1983–85;12:97–101.

Chapter 14: Few Families Are Traditional

Adams RA, Gordon C, Spangler AA. Maternal stress in caring for children with feeding disabilities: implications for health care providers. *J Am Diet Assoc*. 1999;99:962–6.

Ayyangar R. Healthy maintenance and management in childhood disability. *Phys Med Rehabil Clin N Am*. 2002;13:793–821.

Baumrind D. Effects of authoritative control on child behavior. *Child Dev*. 1966;37:887–907.

Case-Smith J. Parenting a child with a chronic medical condition. *Am J Occup Ther*. 2004;58:551–60.

Crawford PB, Gosliner W, Anderson C, Strode P, Becerra-Jones Y, Samuel S, Carroll AM, Ritchie LD. Counseling Latina mothers of preschool children about weight issues: suggestions for a new framework. *J Am Diet Assoc*. 2004;104:387–94.

Cummings EM, Goeke-Morey MC, Papp LM, Dukewich TL. Children's responses to mothers' and fathers' emotionality and tactics in marital conflict in the home. *J Fam Psychol*. 2002;16:478–92.

Eisenberg ME, Olson RE, Neumark-Sztainer D, Story M, Bearinger LH. Correlations between family meals and psychosocial well-being among adolescents. *Arch Pediatr Adolesc Med*. 2004;158:792–6.

Elder JH, Valcante G, Yarandi H, White D, Elder TH. Evaluating in-home training for fathers of children with autism using single-subject experimentation and group analysis methods. *Nurs Res*. 2005;54:22–32.

Family pediatrics report of the Task Force on the Family. *Pediatrics*. 2003;111: 1541–71.

Federal Interagency Forum on Child and Family Statistics. *America's Children: Key National Indicators of Well-Being*. Washington, DC: US Government Printing Office, 1999.

Ford-Gilboe M. Family strengths, motivation, and resources as predictors of health promotion behavior in single-parent and two-parent families. *Res Nurs Health*. 1997;20:205–17.

Gillman MW, Rifas-Shiman SL, Frazier AL, Rockett HR, Carmargo CA Jr, Field AE, Berkey CS, Colditz GA. Family dinner and diet quality among older children and adolescents. *Arch Fam Med*. 2000;9:235–40.

Green SE. "What do you mean 'what's wrong with her?'": stigma and the lives of families of children with disabilities. *Soc Sci Med*. 2003;57:1361–74.

Kelly JB. Marital conflict, divorce, and children's adjustment. *Child Adolesc Psychiatr Clin N Am*. 1998;7:259–71.

Lobato DJ, Kao BT. Integrated sibling-parent group intervention to improve sibling knowledge and adjustment to chronic illness and disability. *J Pediatr Psychol*. 2002;27:711–6.

McLanahan S, Sandfur G. *Growing up with a Single Parent: What Hurts, What Helps*. Cambridge, MA: Harvard University Press, 1994.

Patrick H, Nicklas TA, Hughes SO, Morales M. The benefits of authoritative feeding style: caregiver feeding styles and children's food consumption patterns. *Appetite*. 2005;44:243–9.

Rippe JM, Price JM, Hess SA, Kline G, DeMers KA, Damitz S, Kreidieh I, Freedson P. Improved psychological well-being, quality of life, and health practices in moderately overweight women participating in a 12-week structured weight loss program. *Obes Res*. 1998;6:208–18.

Ritchie LD, Welk G, Styne D, Gerstein DE, Crawford PB. Family environment and pediatric overweight: what is a parent to do? *J Am Diet Assoc*. 2005;105:S70–9.

Shunk JA, Birch LL. Validity of dietary restraint among 5- to 9-year-old girls. *Appetite*. 2004;42:241–7.

Simons RL, Lin K-H, Gordon LC, Conger RD, Lorenz FO. Explaining the higher incidence of adjustment problems among children of divorce compared with those in two-parent families. *J Marriage Fam*. 1999;61:1020–33.

Spieker SJ, Larson NC, Lewis SM, Keller TE, Gilcrist L. Developmental trajectories of disruptive behavior problems in preschool children of adolescent mothers. *Child Dev*. 1999;70:443–58.

Troxel WM, Matthews KA. What are the costs of marital conflict and dissolution of children's physical health? *Clin Child Fam Psychol Rev*. 2004;7:29–57.

Videon TM, Manning CK. Influences on adolescent eating patterns: the importance of family meals. *J Adolesc Health*. 2003;32:365–73.

Williams PD, Williams AR, Graff JC, Hanson S, Stanton A, Hafeman C, Liebergen A, Leuenberg K, Setter RK, Ridder L, Curry H, Barnard M, Sanders S. Interrelationships among variables affecting well siblings and mothers in families of children with a chronic illness or disability. *J Behav Med*. 2002;25:411–24.

Chapter 15: When and Where to Get Extra Help

Atkinson RL, Nitzke SA. School based programmes on obesity. *BMJ*. 2001;323:1018–9.

Austin SB, Field AE, Wiecha J, Peterson KE, Gortmaker SL. The impact of a school-based obesity prevention trial on disordered weight-control behaviors in early adolescent girls. *Arch Pediatr Adolesc Med*. 2005;159:225–30.

Berkowitz RK, Wadden TA, Tershakovec AM, Cronquist JL. Behavior therapy and sibutramine for the treatment of adolescent obesity: a randomized clinical trial. *JAMA*. 2003;289:1805–12.

Bray GA. Drug treatment of obesity. *Rev Endocr Metab Disord*. 2001; 2:403–18.

Bray GA, Blackburn GL, Ferguson JM, Greenway FL, Jain AK, Mendel CM, Mendels J, Ryan DH, Schwartz SL, Scheinbaum ML, Seaton TB. Sibutramine produces dose-related weight loss. *Obes Res*. 1999;7:189–98.

Chanoine JP, Hampl S, Jensen C, Boldrin M, Hauptman J. Effect of orlistat on weight and body composition in obese adolescents: a randomized controlled trial. *JAMA*. 2005;293:2873–83.

Daniels SR, Arnett DK, Eckel RH, Gidding SS, Hayman LL, Kumanyika S, Robinson TN, Scott BJ, St. Jeor S, Williams CL. Overweight in children and adolescents: pathophysiology, consequences, prevention, and treatment. *Circulation*. 2005;111:1999–2012.

Davidson MH, Hauptman J, DiGirolamo M, Foreyt JP, Halsted CH, Heber D, Heimburger DC, Lucas CP, Robbins DC, Chung J, Heymsfield SB. Weight control and risk factor reduction in obese subjects treated for 2 years with orlistat: a randomized controlled trial. *JAMA*. 1999;281:235–42.

Flodmark C-E, Lissau I, Moreno LA, Pietrobelli A, Widhalm K. New insights into the field of children and adolescents' obesity. *Int J Obes*. 2004;28:1189–96.

Fowler-Brown A, Kahwati L. Prevention and treatment of overweight in children and adolescents. *Am Fam Physician*. 2004;69:2591–8.

Inge TH, Lawson L. Treatment considerations for severe adolescent obesity. *Surg Obes Rel Dis*. 2005;1:133–9.

Institute of Medicine. *Weighing the Options: Criteria for Evaluating Weight-Management Programs*. Washington, DC: National Academies Press, 1995.

Institute of Medicine of the National Academies. *Preventing Childhood Obesity: Health in the Balance*. Washington, DC: The National Academies Press, 2005.

Kirk S, Scott B, Daniels S. Pediatric obesity epidemic: treatment options. *J Am Diet Assoc*. 2005;105:S44–51.

Lumeng JC, Gannon K, Appugliese D, Cabral HJ, Zuckerman B. Preschool child care and risk of overweight in 6- to 12-year-old children. *Int J Obes Relat Metab Disord*. 2005;29:60–6.

McDuffe JR, Calis KA, Booth SL, Uwaifo GI, Yanovski JA. Effects of orlistat on fat-soluble vitamins in obese adolescents. *Pharmacotherapy.* 2002;22:814–22.

Muller MJ, Asbeck I, Mast M, Langnase K, Grund A. Prevention of obesity— more than an intention: concept and first results of the Kiel Obesity Prevention Study (KOPS). *Int J Obes Relat Metab Disord.* 2001;25:S66–74.

Pate RR, Trost SG, Mullis R, Sallis JF, Wechsler H, Brown DR. Community interventions to promote proper nutrition and physical activity among youth. *Prev Med.* 2000;31:S138–48.

Veugelers PJ, Fitzgerald AL. Effectiveness of school programs in preventing childhood obesity: a multilevel comparison. *Am J Public Health.* 2005;95:432–5.

Yin Z, Hanes J Jr, Moore JB, Humbles P, Barbeau P, Gutin B. An after-school physical activity program for obesity prevention in children: the Medical College of Georgia FitKid Project. *Eval Health Prof.* 2005;28:67–89.

Index

Page numbers in *italics* refer to photographs.